THE EVERYTHING
HEALTH GUIDE TO
Addiction and Recovery

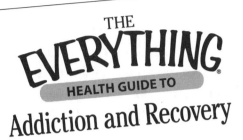

Dear Reader,

I cannot imagine that there is anyone who hasn't been touched by addictions in some way. It is unavoidable in our current society. We now know that the struggle with addictions is not simply due to a lack of willpower or a moral failure. Addictions are complicated and involve our minds, brains, spirits, and environments. Although it is true that many individuals and families have been seriously damaged by addictions, it is also true that the process of recovery can build strength and character. Addictions may bring to light underlying problems that have plagued individuals and families for years. From that perspective, addictions can become a catalyst for "cleaning house," motivating people toward a life of health previously unknown. Patience, kindness, understanding, and grace are key elements for a successful and rewarding outcome. It is my hope that this book will be informative, provide rationales for increasing understanding, and give practical help as you travel the journey of addictions to recovery.

Linda L. Simmons, Psy.D.

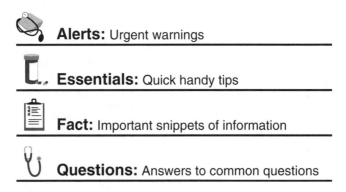

THE

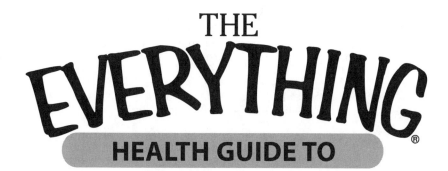

EVERYTHING®

HEALTH GUIDE TO

ADDICTION
AND
RECOVERY

Control your behavior and
build a better life

Linda L. Simmons, Psy.D.

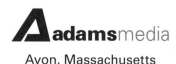

Avon, Massachusetts

*To my parents, Rollie and Cleta Frazier, who have been a constant
source of support, love, and encouragement. Thank you!*

• • •

An Everything® Series Book.
Everything® and everything.com® are registered
trademarks of F+W Publications, Inc.

Published by Adams Media, an F+W Publications Company
57 Littlefield Street, Avon, MA 02322 U.S.A.
www.adamsmedia.com

ISBN 10: 1-59869-806-0
ISBN 13: 978-1-59869-806-0

Printed in Canada.

J I H G F E D C B A

Library of Congress Cataloging-in-Publication Data
is available from the publisher.

This publication is designed to provide accurate and authoritative information
with regard to the subject matter covered. It is sold with the understanding that
the publisher is not engaged in rendering legal, accounting, or other professional advice. If legal advice or other expert assistance is required, the services
of a competent professional person should be sought.
—From a *Declaration of Principles* jointly adopted by a Committee of the
American Bar Association and a Committee of Publishers and Associations

Many of the designations used by manufacturers and sellers to distinguish their
products are claimed as trademarks. Where those designations appear in this
book and Adams Media was aware of a trademark claim, the designations have
been printed with initial capital letters.

The Everything® Health Guide to Addiction and Recovery is intended as a reference volume only, not as a medical manual. In light of the complex, individual,
and specific nature of health problems, this book is not intended to replace
professional medical advice. The ideas, procedures, and suggestions in this
book are intended to supplement, not replace, the advice of a trained medical
professional. Consult your physician before adopting the suggestions in this
book, as well as about any condition that may require diagnosis or medical
attention. The author and publisher disclaim any liability arising directly or
indirectly from the use of this book.

*This book is available at quantity discounts for bulk purchases.
For information, please call 1-800-289-0963.*

*All the examples and dialogues used in this book are fictional and have
been created by the author to illustrate medical situations.*

Contents

Introduction   xi

Chapter 1:   **The Nature of Addiction**   1
Abuse Versus Dependence   1
How Addiction Works in the Brain   6
Effects on Other Biological Systems   7
Emotional Effects of Addiction   8
Psychological Effects of Addiction   10

Chapter 2:   **Identifying Addiction**   15
Risk Factors   15
Symptoms   19
When the Line Has Been Crossed   21
Self-Evaluation   21
Recognizing Addictive Behaviors   23
Denial   25

Chapter 3:   **What Causes Addiction?**   27
The Question of Willpower   27
Genetic Factors   28
Biological Factors   30
Environmental Factors   31
Family Relations and Learned Behavior   33
Psychological Factors   35
An Addictive Personality   37

Chapter 4:   **Cultural Lures and Addiction**   39
Advertising Is Everywhere   39
Why Advertising Is So Effective   40
The Curiosity Factor   41
Peer Pressure and Social Expectations   43
Influence by Celebrities   44
Ethnic and Cultural Differences   46
Dealing with External Pressures   47
Seeking Help   48

Chapter 5: **Alcohol Addiction**   **49**
            What Is Alcoholism?   49
            The "Social Drinker"   54
            The Effects of Alcohol on Moods   56
            How Alcohol Affects Women Versus Men   57
            Reading the Signs and Symptoms   59
            Talking to a Loved One about His or Her Problem   60
            The Road to Recovery   61
            Choosing to Take the Twelve Steps   62
            The Myth of the "Dry Drunk"   63

Chapter 6: **Substance Addiction**   **65**
            Introduction to Drugs   65
            Common Substances of Abuse   70
            How the Body Reacts   72
            Knowing the Signs and Symptoms   74
            The Criminal Element   75
            Talking to a Loved One about His or Her Problem   76
            Overcoming Substance Addiction   78
            Rehab and Recovery   79

Chapter 7: **Nicotine Addiction**   **81**
            Got a Light?   81
            The Physiological Effects of Nicotine   84
            The Psychological Component   87
            The Dangers of Secondhand Smoke   88
            The Most Difficult Addiction to Break?   89
            Talking to a Loved One about His or Her Problem   90
            Treatment Options   91

Chapter 8: **Prescription Drug Addiction**   **95**
            But the Doctor Prescribed It!   95
            When the Risks Outweigh the Benefits   96
            Commonly Abused Prescription Drugs   100
            Drastic Measures to Get Drugs   104
            Talking to a Loved One about His or Her Problem   105
            Getting Help   106

Chapter 9: **Food Addiction**   **108**
            When Food Becomes More than Nutrition   108
            Signs of Food Addiction   109
            Behavioral Contributions to Food Addiction   109
            Societal Pressure   111
            Are All Foods Addictive?   112

The Lure of the Drive-Through Window   115
Talking to a Loved One about His or Her Problem   116
Treatment Options   118

Chapter 10: Behavioral Addictions   120
When Does a Hobby Become an Addiction?   120
Impulsive Behavior Versus Addiction   121
Shopping/Spending Addiction   123
Exercise Addiction   126
Other Behavioral Addictions   129
Effects on Family Members   133
Talking to a Loved One about His or Her Problem   134
Seeking Help   134

Chapter 11: Gambling Addiction   136
It's Just Entertainment!   136
Watch for the Signs   140
Gambling Is Good for the Economy, Right?   141
Internet Gambling   144
The Effects on Families Are Not Fun   144
Confronting the Game   145
Treatment Options   146

Chapter 12: Relational Addictions   148
Love Addiction   148
Serial Dating   153
Sex Addiction   154
Relationships from a Distance: Cybersex   157
Chat Room Addiction   159
The Danger of Relational Addictions   160
Talking to a Loved One about His or Her Problem   160
Seeking Help   161

Chapter 13: Pornography Addiction   163
Don't All Men Like to Look?   163
Entertainment or Addiction?   165
The Effects of Pornography on Relationships   168
Legal Implications   170
Treatment for the Addict   171
Support for Partners of Pornography Addicts   173

Chapter 14: Technology and Addiction — 174

The New Complication in Addictions — 174
Video Game Addiction — 177
Addiction to Cell Phones and Other Technological
    Devices — 180
Internet Addiction — 182
The Lure of Anonymity — 184
Talking to a Loved One about His or Her Problem — 185
Seeking Help — 186

Chapter 15: Roadblocks to Treatment — 188

Dealing with Denial — 188
Budgeting for Treatment — 191
Finding the Right Treatment for You — 194
Locating Qualified Professionals — 197
What if Treatment Threatens My Job? — 198
Talking to Friends and Family about Treatment — 199
Getting Support — 200

Chapter 16: Additional Treatment Options — 201

Detoxification — 201
Medications Used in Addiction and Recovery — 203
Alternative Treatment Options — 209
Faith-Based Treatment Programs — 216
The Risks of Treatment — 217

Chapter 17: Recovery — 218

Become Knowledgeable about Recovery — 218
Changing Thinking Patterns — 219
Technological Aids — 222
Avoiding Relapse — 224
Effective Use of Support Systems — 226
Utilizing Community Resources — 228
The Face of Healthy Recovery — 229

Chapter 18: Relapse Prevention — 231

Be Prepared — 231
Recognizing Triggers — 235
Managing—and Recovering from—Slips — 236
Be Aware of High-Risk Situations — 237
Evaluating Relationships — 239
Developing Healthy Self-Esteem — 240
Keep the Support Going! — 241

Chapter 19: Real-Life Considerations   243
Someone Has to Pay the Bills   243
Who's Going to Take Out the Trash?   249
Maintaining Healthy Relationships   251
Effective Time Management   252
You Can Be a Good Parent and Help Yourself   256
Restoring Credibility in the Community   257

Chapter 20: How Addictions Affect Family Members   259
Damaged Family Bonds   259
Dealing with Difficult Emotions   261
Communication Is Key   263
Constructive Fighting   265
When Roles Are Reversed   267
The Effects of Financial Hardships   270
Rebuilding Trust   271
Establishing New and Healthy Family Relationships   272

Chapter 21: Hope for a Balanced Life   274
The Mind-Body-Spirit Connection   274
Good Self-Care   275
Personal Growth   278
Meaningful Work and Passionate Play   279
Making Room for Therapy   281
Developing Satisfying Relationships   282
Leave the Past Behind and Look to the Future   283

Appendix A   285

Appendix B   291

Index   300

Acknowledgments

I'd like to thank Janice Pieroni, my agent, for her editing advice, advocacy, perseverance, encouragement, and, most of all, friendship. I also have great appreciation for my husband, Chuck, who kept the home front going so I could write. Appreciation goes to the staff at Adams Media who gave me the opportunity to work on this worthwhile project. Finally, I would like to thank Sam, Adam, Debbie, and Doug for their faithful support and belief in me.

Introduction

SADLY, ADDICTIONS ARE front-page news every day. No one is immune from either having an addiction or being affected by someone else's addiction. Addictions damage one's health, self-image, career, and relationships. Resulting financial, medical, and legal problems are common and serious. Historically, individuals with addictions were laughed at, ignored, or shunned. It was thought that addictions were due to a lack of self-discipline and/or to moral failure. Addictions have become too costly in many ways to be ignored anymore. Research has demonstrated that brain chemistry and functioning plus the body's physiological reactions to addictions make self-discipline extremely difficult. Although moral, healthy choices may help someone manage his addiction, they cannot change anyone's brain.

The pressures and inventions of modern life have contributed to the expansion of addictions. Technology has created a whole new venue for addictive disorders. Science has shown that even compulsive behaviors such as gambling, shopping, and Internet use can activate addictive responses in one's brain. "Designer drugs" have increased the selection of addictive substances, and they are more potent and dangerous than ever before. Social and peer pressure have drastically lowered the age at which addictions begin. Preteens and teenagers are the fastest-growing population to succumb to addictions. This age group is the least capable, biologically, of making rational and wise decisions regarding addictions. Families, teachers, and friends must rise to the occasion to help kids get through these growing-up years safely. Supervision, education, and good role-modeling will go a long way toward curbing the tide of addictions in our youth.

The good news is that more treatments for addiction exist now than ever before in history. The stigma once associated with receiving treatment is disappearing as friends, family, and employers realize the great cost of untreated addictions. It is now recognized that many individuals with addictions also have co-occurring mental health disorders. Of course, this complicates the whole picture of addictions. Individuals with a dual diagnosis need to be treated for both disorders simultaneously for recovery to be successful. There are a plethora of medications now available to treat both the addictions and the mental health disorders. This is very exciting—addicted individuals who have suffered for years are now finding relief and hope.

Support groups for both addicted individuals and families are in existence in almost every community. Whether these groups are twelve-step programs, faith-based programs, mental health support groups, or Internet groups, something is available to meet the needs of any addict. Support groups are wonderful, in that they have sprung up out of recognition of and respect for the power of addictions. It is a rare person who can successfully recover from an entrenched addiction on her own. There are more and more professionals available who have received specialized training in working with addicted persons and family members affected by addictions. This means that an addict will be treated with respect, empathy, and interventions more carefully designed to target her unique needs. Specialized treatment centers designed to treat addictions and dual disorders provide state-of-the-art inpatient and residential services. Although technology has created many problems in the area of addictions, it has also provided many helps. Unbelievable amounts of resources and educational material can be accessed through the Internet. Twenty-four hours a day, seven days a week, an addict can access online support groups, hear encouraging messages on addiction topics, and interact with other addicts who are struggling in similar ways. There is every reason for an addict, her friends, and her family members to be hopeful. A celebration of recovery lies ahead!

CHAPTER 1

The Nature of Addiction

THERE ARE MANY kinds of addictions. Some people are addicted to drugs or alcohol. Others are addicted to gambling, food, pornography, or playing games on the Internet. What addictions have in common is their tendency to take over a person's life. Once substance use or behaviors rise to the level of addiction, they can be very difficult to manage. Treatment and recovery can be extremely challenging and often expensive. But there is hope. In spite of the difficulty, people can and do recover from addictions. If you or someone you care about is struggling with addictions, recovery is possible!

Abuse Versus Dependence

With respect to addictions, is there a difference between abuse and dependence? This is a commonly asked question; the answer is yes. It is an important distinction to understand, as it may affect the type of treatment sought out and the level of difficulty encountered in recovery. Although both abuse and dependence can cause significant problems in a person's life, dependence involves physiological changes that lead to an addictive process. Therefore, dependence on substances and/or behaviors can be more difficult and complicated to treat. Repeated abuse of substances and/or behaviors can develop into habits that are hard to break. However, abuse doesn't necessarily lead into the physiological changes of addiction. Either abusing or being dependent upon a substance or a behavior can diminish one's ability to fully participate in and enjoy everyday life.

Substance Abuse

Substance abuse occurs when a person uses drugs or consumes alcohol excessively. This excessive use typically causes significant problems in a person's life. For example, if a person drinks excessively on a Sunday evening and is unable to go to work on Monday morning or is unable to perform job functions as well as usual, this is abuse. It is abuse when a person uses alcohol or other substances excessively and then gets in his car to drive home, putting his own and others' lives in danger. There may be legal problems such as DUIs (driving under the influence) or arrests for disturbing the peace as a result of excessive use of alcohol or other substances. A parent who uses alcohol or other substances excessively may not be able to take care of her children responsibly. Essential household functions such as taking out the trash, maintaining cleanliness, and so forth may be neglected when men and women use substances excessively. Persons who are abusing substances often repeatedly have problems getting along with others. These are only a few illustrations of the ways in which substance abuse can negatively affect a person's everyday life.

Alert

How big of a concern is substance abuse and dependency? The U.S. Substance Abuse and Mental Health Services Administration (SAMHSA) reported in its 2006 National Survey on Drug Use and Health that 22.6 million individuals aged twelve and older experienced either substance abuse or dependency problems in the previous year. This is approximately 9.2 percent of the U.S. population.

Historically, it has been more common for substance abuse to be associated with men, but times have changed. Both men and women are now seen engaging in substance abuse or addictive behaviors in movies, commercials, and advertisements. For some, substance abuse may be considered a rite of passage or an introduction into an adult social arena considered by a certain segment of the population as acceptable entertainment. One might think that with more openness related to substance abuse in our culture, it would be easier to acknowledge the problems and get treatment. Sadly, however, shame is still a significant barrier to overcome in recognizing substance abuse and seeking treatment. This is especially true if the problems and negative consequences associated with substance abuse become public. Confusion and mixed messages abound.

Essential

It is now commonly accepted that all substance-related and behavioral addictions involve compulsive use, loss of control, and continued use despite adverse consequences. These are important characteristics for you to be aware of as you consider whether you or someone you care about may have a problem with addictions.

Substance Dependence

Dependence on a substance can include any or all of the problems of substance abuse. It is important to be aware, however, that with dependence, the problems become even more complicated because of the physiological changes that occur. A couple of key points that will be important to understand involve the two primary physiological issues associated with dependence: tolerance and withdrawal. Tolerance means a person needs more and more of the substance over time to get the same effects he experienced when he first began using the substance. It can also mean that if a person's use of the substance stays the same, the initial effects experienced will decrease with use over time. Say, for example, that a person had her first beer at sixteen and got a real buzz from the experience. By the time she is twenty, she might need six to twelve beers to get that same buzz. If she is a regular drinker and keeps her drinking level to one beer, she would likely feel no buzz at all by age twenty. (Of course, this time frame would vary for the occasional drinker versus the regular drinker.)

 Question

Can alcoholism develop if someone only drinks wine or beer?
Yes. Since wine and beer have lower alcohol content than other alcoholic beverages, some mistakenly believe that they cannot develop an addiction. The fact is, if enough wine and beer are consumed, alcohol addiction can develop.

After a person has used an addictive substance over a period of time, he may experience withdrawal symptoms if he chooses to stop using the substance. Withdrawal symptoms can be physical, behavioral, or psychological in nature. The symptoms that a person deals with are specific to the substance being used. For example, the withdrawal symptoms of alcohol are not completely the same as those of cocaine usage. More will be discussed later on the unique withdrawal symptoms of different substances.

No one would argue that withdrawal symptoms for any substance can be very uncomfortable, unpleasant, and even life-threatening. An addict in recovery goes through an ambivalent struggle knowing that taking more of the addictive substance would result in relief from the discomfort of withdrawal. This can lead to misunderstanding by those who might see the addict as insincere and untrustworthy, saying she wants to be rid of her addiction but not following through with the necessary treatment to achieve her goal. In many cases, it's not that the addict doesn't want recovery, it's that she is avoiding the pain of withdrawal. This is the time when an addict needs to be patient with herself and most needs the understanding and support of her friends, family, and treatment providers.

Fact

Addictions were first identified as a disease process rather than a mental disorder or moral failure by Dr. Benjamin Rush in 1810. In 1945 the American Medical Association formally adopted this definition as well, and most other professional organizations have followed its lead.

It is not uncommon for an individual to take more of a substance than was originally intended. This may be due to peer pressure, not realizing the potency of the substance, or experimental use gone awry. He might find himself wanting to stop using the substance but repeatedly being unsuccessful. This is very discouraging, and people in this situation need a great deal of support to succeed. In such circumstances, the addicted person may realize that more and more of his time and money are being spent on getting the substance. He may give up other activities, even activities he typically enjoys, in favor of using the substance. He may also find himself continuing to use the substance in spite of the knowledge that there will be serious consequences that can negatively affect him and people he loves.

Essential

The biological processes of tolerance and withdrawal have been found to occur in both substance addiction and addictions to compulsive behaviors such as gambling, pornography, sex addictions, food addiction, compulsive spending, and other excessive behaviors. The technical term for these biological processes is *neuroadaptation*.

How Addiction Works in the Brain

It is now believed that all types of frequently abused substances set off a pleasure circuit in the brain. The same pleasure circuit works for alcohol, amphetamines, chocolate, sugar, sex, and so forth. According to *The Owner's Manual for the Brain* by Dr. Pierce Howard, this pleasure circuit begins in the amygdala of the brain, then travels to the anterior cingulum, and finally on to the temporal lobes. As a whole, the pleasure circuit is called the median forebrain bundle, or in lay language, the "hedonic highway" or "pleasure pathway."

 Fact

Cravings can be triggered by damage to the delivery system that moves dopamine from one brain cell (neuron) to the next. Many addicts report they often use substances not to feel "high," but to feel "normal." Their goal is to stop the cravings, and at this point, the survival process begins for the addict.

Neurotransmitters are chemicals in the brain that transmit messages from one brain cell (neuron) to another. Dopamine, one such neurotransmitter, is the chemical most involved in the pleasure circuit and so is linked with addiction. All substances of addiction interfere with the normal reabsorption of dopamine by neurons in the brain. By preventing this reabsorption, high levels of dopamine remain in the gaps between the neurons. Since one of the primary functions of dopamine is to give a person a sensation of pleasure, these excessive amounts of dopamine give an individual the "high" sensation. The dopamine receptor cell is the one type of cell found all along the "pleasure pathway."

Another interesting fact in this process concerns a space between neurons in the brain called the *synaptic gap*. Ordinarily, neurotransmitters such as dopamine only stay in this space long enough to get picked up by receptor sites in the next neuron and then they get passed along to be used in their normal manner. However, as mentioned, when absorption by the receptor sites of the next neuron is blocked, the dopamine, for example, stays in the synaptic gap and the person then experiences a "high" or pleasure effect. Many substances, such as cocaine, amphetamines, Ritalin, nicotine, and marijuana, block the absorption of dopamine by neurons in the brain. When addictive substances are used repeatedly, it is thought to damage the dopamine delivery system, the normal movement of dopamine from one neuron to the next. Many believe that once addictions have damaged this dopamine pleasure circuit, it never completely returns to normal.

Effects on Other Biological Systems

Although the brain is the primary biological system affected by addictions, the rest of the body can be affected as well. Addictions have been connected with lung disease, cardiovascular disease, stroke, cancer, obesity, HIV/AIDS, and nerve cell damage in the peripheral nervous system. Different abused substances affect different biological systems. Inhalants, for instance, are toxic substances found in common household products. They are readily available and inexpensive. Examples of inhalants include oven cleaner, gasoline, glue, spray paints, and other aerosols. The intoxicating vapors of inhalants can be sniffed, breathed in, or sprayed directly into the mouth or nose. They can damage the heart, lungs, and brain. Heart failure and death can occur in a single instance of sniffing an inhalant. If you are the parent of an elementary-school child, you need to know that inhalants are often the first substance that children use experimentally because they are so easily accessible. Therefore, it is important to keep all inhalants in a safe place, educate your children on the dangers associated with these substances, and provide adequate supervision. These simple measures can help your family avert a needless tragedy. Inhalants are a dramatic example, but most other abused substances also cause serious damage to major biological systems. As if this information were not worrisome enough, consider also that many individuals who abuse substances have multiple addictions. The interaction effects of using multiple drugs simultaneously present phenomenal risks for the addict.

Alert

> Secondhand tobacco smoke has been the subject of much heated discussion. According to the Surgeon General's 2006 report "The Health Consequences of Involuntary Exposure to Tobacco Smoke," environmental smoke increases the risk of heart disease by 25 to 30 percent and lung cancer by 20 to 30 percent in individuals who have never smoked.

Other issues to consider are the biological effects of addictions that may occur indirectly and that can reach beyond the addict himself. The harm to nonsmokers caused by environmental smoke has prompted legislation around the world limiting smoking to designated areas to protect nonsmokers. At times, addicts turn to criminal activity and prostitution out of desperation to obtain their substance(s) of choice; innocent bystanders as well as the addict may be endangered. Addicts who share intravenous needles and/or who engage in unprotected sexual activity may infect themselves or others with HIV/AIDS. Addicts who practice poor hygiene and neglect general good health practices are at risk for infections and malnutrition, with their accompanying biological maladies.

Emotional Effects of Addiction

Psychoanalysts in the 1960s came up with the notion that people often used addictive substances to medicate themselves when experiencing emotional pain. In subsequent years, many others have come to agree with this theory. Because of the pleasure pathway that addictive substances and behaviors can activate, the addict may initially feel relief.

Those very painful emotions that a person might try to numb or soothe with substances or compulsive behaviors may actually become intensified as time goes on. For example, if a man has a flask of alcohol hidden in his desk drawer at work to calm his nerves before an important presentation, imagine the anxiety of fearing he will lose his job if he's caught. Or consider the woman who hides her feelings of loneliness with compulsive shopping. There might be a false sense of camaraderie gained from being in a crowded mall and conversing with salesclerks over purchases. However, the worry, fear, and shame of being discovered create a prison of loneliness for her that won't go away with unfulfilling purchases.

 Question

What is anhedonia?
Anhedonia is the inability to experience pleasure as one once did. Feelings become blunted and flat. Substance abuse and dependence can lead to anhedonia as the brain's pleasure circuit is damaged. An addict will often increase her substance use to try to regain her ability to experience pleasure and enjoy life.

Anger is another powerful emotion that often accompanies addictions. There are many possible sources of anger in this situation. An addict may perceive that life has treated him unfairly after experiencing a job loss, divorce, or financial setbacks, and use addictive substances or behaviors to try to soothe his anger. Anger may serve to keep others away so the addict can use substances privately. You may well understand through your own experience that there are almost always other emotions beneath the anger. Common underlying emotions are fear, disappointment, and hurt. An addict may fear that she will not be able to live up to the expectations of others. She may feel disappointed that life has not gone the direction she wanted. Hurts inflicted by others, whether they are physical, emotional, or psychological, may be hard to manage and subsequently treated with addictive substances or behaviors.

Psychological Effects of Addiction

Addictions often affect or change the way a person thinks about things. Your thoughts, or cognitions, can serve many functions. One is defensiveness. An addict who may not be ready to acknowledge her addiction may feel a need to defend her continued use of addictive substances. One method of doing this is to deny in one's thoughts that the addiction is a problem. Or a person may use his thinking processes to rationalize or explain away his continued use of an addictive substance or behavior in spite of the negative consequences. Thoughts may become obsessive as an addict pursues the use of the addictive substance or behavior to calm the cravings or curb the withdrawal symptoms. Following are some examples that may help you understand how addictions can affect a person's mind and thinking processes.

Denial

Denial is the most common thought process used in dealing with addictions. A college student might try to convince herself and others that cocaine use is just part of college life and that on graduation, she'll easily drop it and move into a successful climb up the career ladder. Once a person becomes addicted, she often denies or ignores the strong hold the addiction has on her life. A father may go downstairs after his wife and children are in bed to view pornography, denying that this is anything more than adult entertainment and that it might negatively affect his marriage. Denial is used by the addict to provide a false sense of security for himself as he tries to convince himself that everything is fine and under control. For friends and loved ones, the addict's denial is very frustrating. From the outside looking in, they can clearly see that very little may be under control for the addict. Confronting an addict's denial may generate a great deal of anger. One of the most common questions asked by those who care about the addict is how to effectively confront and break through denial. Confronting and facing denial requires honesty and courage on the part of the addict and those who care about her. Detailed help on the issue of denial will be addressed later.

Alert

> It is a common myth nowadays that young people will grow out of addictive behaviors. Esther Gwinnell, M.D. and Christine Adamec in their book *The Encyclopedia of Addictions and Addictive Behaviors* assert that addictive behaviors that begin in early and mid-adolescence typically have long-term effects into adulthood.

Obsessive Thinking

Obsessive thinking is thinking focused entirely on a specific object—in this case, an addictive substance or behavior. In the obsessive-thinking mode, the addictive substance or behavior is in the driver's seat and determines the direction of the driver's life. The addiction dictates how the person spends his time and money, who he hangs out with socially, what he has to do to obtain more of the substance, and the excuses he has to make to cover up the obsession. All resources are directed toward obtaining the object of the obsession, which is the addictive substance or behavior. Obsessive thinking can shut out other thoughts that one should pay attention to—for example, paying one's bills in a timely manner or getting the kids to school on time. In other words, obsessive thoughts can take over one's life.

Grandiose Thinking

Alongside obsessive thinking there is often the companion, grandiose thinking. In simple terms, grandiose thinking conveys the idea "It's all about me!" For the addict indulging in grandiose thinking, nothing is more important in her life than herself and her addiction.

There is a false assumption that others will feel the same and put their own needs aside in deference to the addict. You can imagine the conflicts that arise in the addict's family and social circle when others decide not to support this type of thinking.

 Fact

> The cerebral cortex is the area of our brain involved in thinking, planning, problem-solving, and decision-making. The National Institute on Drug Abuse asserts that chronic exposure to drugs of abuse causes disruptions in the brain that negatively affect a person's ability to make sound decisions. At the same time, the brain's drive to take drugs increases.

Thought Distortions

Thought distortions are those thoughts that may contain an element of truth but also contain misinformation or exaggerated information. Thought distortions typically include all-or-nothing, black-or-white thinking, and lack the perspective that there may be some truth between the extremes. For instance, an alcoholic might have a successful treatment experience but six months later, relapse. Rather than seeing this simply as one slip on the road to full recovery, if she was engaging in distorted thinking, she might see herself as a complete failure who doesn't have a chance at beating the addiction. Another example might be a man who was fired from his job because of his boss finding pornography on a business computer. Distorted thinking would be that everyone in the industry will likely know about his pornography addiction now and he'll never be able to find work in his field again. The truth is that, with treatment, many employers would likely give him a second chance if he had the job skills they were seeking. Distorted thinking needs to be firmly and lovingly challenged in order to help the addict restore his thinking to a realistic perspective of himself and the world around him.

Learning and Memory

The cerebral cortex, amygdala, and hippocampus are areas of the brain involved in learning and memory. Addictions also affect these structures. It is important to know that many of the same brain pathways that involve addictive processes are also responsible for learning and memory. Memories are affected by addictions in two ways. First, addictions alter the neurological connections in the brain and thus negatively affect learning and memory. Secondly, behavioral connections made between the addictive substance and pleasurable responses are laid down in memory. When reminders of those pleasurable reinforcers are encountered in the environment, memories are recalled and lure the addict to crave her substance yet again. This is a very frustrating experience for an addicted individual who is fighting for recovery. It is very difficult for her to put these memories of pleasurable responses behind her so she can move forward to a clean and sober life. It is also frustrating and discouraging when an addicted person discovers that his capacity to learn and remember things has suffered. Understanding and patience is called for as someone with addictions fights to defeat these battles of the mind.

 Question

What is Korsakoff's syndrome?

Korsakoff's syndrome is a memory disorder commonly caused by a thiamine deficiency associated with alcoholism. Individuals who drink excessive amounts of alcohol often neglect healthy nutrition, and multiple vitamin deficiencies develop. In Korsakoff's syndrome, a person may remember minute details of her past, but be unable to recall what she had for breakfast.

Cognitive functioning, or the capacity of the brain to think, reason, remember, and make decisions, is affected by another neurotransmitter called *glutamate*. Glutamate also has influence on the pleasure circuit in the brain, though not as significantly as dopamine. It is also thought that glutamate helps one access the pleasurable memories of substance abuse "highs." This function of glutamate is related to an addict's tendency to relapse because these pleasurable memories lead to drug-seeking behavior. When the brain's concentration of glutamate is changed through substance abuse and the absorption of glutamate is reduced, memory and learning functions are negatively affected. Again, it seems that once this type of damage occurs in the brain, the effects are extensive and long-term. As one can see, addictions affect a person's entire physical, emotional, and psychological being. The more these effects and interactions are understood, the more one will be able to engage in successful recovery or help a loved one.

CHAPTER 2

Identifying Addiction

ADDICTION IN GENERAL has been described as a compulsive craving for something in spite of negative consequences that come from pursuing its use. The compulsive cravings of addiction have physiological, psychological, and emotional components. Traditionally, the notion of addictions has been connected with cocaine, alcohol, heroin, nicotine, and other chemically based substances. Current thinking is that there are certain compulsive behaviors—including gambling, shopping, eating, and watching pornography—that can set off similar addictive responses in the brain.

Risk Factors

An addictive risk factor is anything that might increase the likelihood of becoming involved with an addictive substance or behavior. Risk factors can be biological, social, emotional, or environmental in nature. For a long time now, it has been noted that certain addictions, particularly alcoholism, seem to run in families. Scientists currently believe that there are several genes associated with addiction. Genetic research related to addictions will undoubtedly contribute greatly to more specific and effective treatments as further information is gained about the genes involved in the addictive process. Does this mean that everyone born to parents with addictions will inevitably become addicted? No, it does not. It simply means that there is a greater likelihood of addictions developing when there is a positive family history. Remember, other risk factors also contribute to the development of addiction.

It is important to understand that addictions are not simply bad habits. If a person has developed a bad habit of gossiping, that doesn't mean he is addicted to the behavior of gossiping. Someone who may have gotten into the bad habit of eating two bowls of ice cream every night at bedtime is not necessarily addicted to ice cream. This is an important distinction that needs clarification. A bad habit is a repetitive behavior that someone may engage in, at times without even thinking about it, that may be unhealthy in some way or cause other types of problems. An addiction brings about multiple changes in a person that don't occur in a nonaddict who may use the same substance or behavior.

Essential

Positive family relationships are not only a helpful deterrent in preventing the development of addictions in children and adolescents but also contribute to earlier identification of addiction problems that may have developed. A lack of attachment between children and parents and a lack of parental supervision are contributing factors in the development of addictions in youth.

Social Risk Factors

Young people in particular are significantly influenced by the behaviors of their friends. Developmentally, the teen years are focused on establishing relationships with peers. Too often, if the promise of a friendship or romantic relationship comes with the price tag of joining in risky behaviors that have the potential for addiction, the relationship will win out. Most adults addicted to nicotine began smoking around fourteen years of age with the purpose of fitting in with peers. It has also been observed that when young people are under the influence of drugs and alcohol, they are more likely to commit crimes, assault others, and participate in risky sexual behaviors. This is important information for parents to know. Adequate parental supervision is a key factor in identifying and preventing addictions in young people.

Teenagers are not the only ones susceptible to social pressures when it comes to addictive behaviors. Adults also enjoy the approval and acceptance of their peers, even peers who engage in or encourage addictive behaviors. It can take a lot of strength to turn down a beer while watching a football game with buddies when everyone else is drinking heavily. Similarly, you can imagine the courage it takes for someone addicted to spending to go shopping with friends and say no to sales on the clearance rack.

Alert

The Genetic Science Learning Center at the University of Utah claims that approximately 10 percent of all people who experiment with drugs become addicted. The influence of risk factors, particularly multiple risk factors, is significant in determining the outcome of addictions. Scientists are learning more all the time about the interplay of risk factors.

Environmental Risk Factors of Addiction

Environmental risk factors include a person's connection to her community. If you live in a community with a tolerant attitude toward substance use, firearms, and crime, the risk for addictions is increased. Conversely, attachment and identification to a community situation that does not condone drug use decreases the risk of addiction.

School systems are a significant part of communities. Academic failure, particularly in later elementary years, is a risk factor for addictions because children experiencing low self-esteem due to academic failure may be tempted to turn to substance abuse to manage their damaged emotions or to fit in with substance-abusing peers. Teachers, parents, and the community can have a positive effect on children and decrease the risk of addictions by helping them to be successful academically. A sense of accomplishment academically may eliminate a child's need to use addictive substances to self-medicate depressive or anxious feelings.

Constructive community activities contribute to positive self-esteem and self-confidence in both adults and young people. When such opportunities are lacking and there is a dearth of meaningful things to do with one's time, susceptible people may be at risk for developing addictions. Activating the dopamine pleasure pathway with addictive substances or behaviors can lead a person to feel alive, even though the feelings may be fleeting and the consequences may prove to be destructive.

 Fact

D.A.R.E. (Drug Abuse Resistance Education) is an educational program that was started in 1983 in Los Angeles. Specially trained police officers present educational lessons to children from kindergarten through twelfth grade on how to resist peer pressure, drugs, and violence. This successful program is now being presented in 75 percent of school districts in the United States.

Emotional Risk Factors of Addiction

While emotions such as anxiety, depression, anger, and loneliness may result from the problems surrounding addictions, when these emotions are primary, or pre-existing, they can be risk factors for developing addictions. Some people use illicit drugs as a method of "self-medicating" painful emotions. Illicit drugs are drugs that, even if legal, have not been legitimately prescribed to treat a diagnosed ailment or condition. As mentioned previously, addictions stimulate dopamine production as well as other neurotransmitters, such as serotonin, that give sensations of pleasure and well-being. Therefore, addictions can become a harmful way of coping or covering up emotions that seem too painful or overwhelming to face.

When someone is better able to manage her emotions in constructive and appropriate ways, she is more able to resist the temptation to use addictions to feel better. Sometimes, however, it is not her own emotions that are the problem. As social beings, people are also affected by the emotions of others. It can be very difficult to consistently live or work with another person who may be chronically angry or upset. Fear or anxiety over the negative reactions of others may lead someone to turn toward addictive substances and/or behaviors rather than working things through in a constructive manner. Developing effective problem-solving skills can minimize the risk of using addictions to manage relationship problems.

Alert

> Children who exhibit aggressive behaviors, demonstrate a lack of self-control, and have a difficult temperament may be at greater risk for drug addiction. This is important information for parents to note as they seek to work with their children to prevent and identify the development of addictions.

Symptoms

The symptoms of addiction are many and varied. At first, many signs and symptoms of addiction may seem like overreactions to stressful circumstances. Isolated signs or symptoms may be just that, an overreaction to stressful circumstances. However, when multiple signs and symptoms of addiction begin to appear, it is time to pay attention.

The following behaviors may be indications that someone is at risk for or has developed an addiction:

- Drugs and/or alcohol are seen as necessary components to having fun.
- School attendance suddenly declines, along with performance and grades.
- Items around the house may begin to disappear or he may start to sell prized possessions.

- He may begin to display angry outbursts, mood swings, irritability, manic behavior, or an overall attitude change.
- Others may notice him talking incoherently or making inappropriate remarks in conversations.
- His physical appearance and grooming deteriorate.
- His social circle may change or dwindle to include only those individuals who also use addictive substances or behaviors.
- He may begin to engage in secretive or suspicious behaviors, such as making frequent trips to the restroom, basement, or other isolated areas where drug use or compulsive behaviors would be undisturbed.
- Talk about addiction(s) and pressuring others to use may begin to dominate how he spends his time. Alternatively, someone may consistently experience and express feelings of exhaustion, depression, and hopelessness.

Be aware that these same types of signs and symptoms are true for the behavioral addictions as well. The complexity and all-encompassing nature of addictions may be overwhelming. It is also common for a person to deny or try to explain away the signs and symptoms of addiction. One should not hesitate to consult with a professional if help is needed to sort things out and get an accurate diagnosis.

Essential

Remember that addiction is a chronic disease. Addictions and chronic illnesses such as cardiovascular disease, diabetes, and cancer share many common features. They both tend to have a genetic component and are influenced by environmental factors and behaviors.

Take heart and be encouraged. As with other chronic illnesses, the signs and symptoms of addictions do respond to appropriate treatment. Correctly reading the signs and symptoms of addictions and receiving an accurate diagnosis is the key in choosing treatments that will be effective. There will be additional discussion about treatments later, but in summary, they might include therapy, medications, and long-term lifestyle changes.

When the Line Has Been Crossed

Determining when the use of potentially addictive substances and compulsive behaviors cease to be fun, entertaining, or experimental is the most important step toward identifying the addiction. The line between recreation and addiction is crossed when control is lost. When addictive substances and behaviors take priority over the necessities of life, they are no longer recreation, hobbies, or fun interests. Humans don't function well when addictions take over. It is highly unlikely that anyone would engage in addictive behaviors or substance use with the intent of allowing such behaviors or use to take over her life. Quite often, an addicted person is as surprised as everyone else at the power of the addiction.

Self-Evaluation

It takes tremendous courage to face the possibility of personal addiction. A willingness to ask and answer some difficult questions will be necessary to identify whether you or a loved one has an addiction. Determining that you or a loved one does have an addiction is the first step toward receiving the help needed for you (or her) to overcome it and regain control of your lives. Consider the following questions as you seek to identify the signs and symptoms of addictions.

- ✓ Have you ever wondered if you should cut down on your drinking, smoking, gambling, spending, etc.?
- ✓ Do you become annoyed if others ask you about your substance use or compulsive behaviors?
- ✓ Do you ever feel guilty in relation to your substance use or compulsive behaviors?

✓ Do you feel compelled to use your substance or engage in your compulsive behaviors first thing in the morning?

✓ Have others complained about your substance use or compulsive behaviors and the negative effects they may have experienced as a result?

✓ Have you lost friends as a result of your substance use or compulsive behaviors?

✓ Have you ever experienced legal problems as a result of your substance use or compulsive behaviors?

✓ Have you ever lost a job or received disciplinary action at work because of substance use or compulsive behaviors?

✓ Have you ever wondered if you should seek professional help for your substance use or compulsive behaviors?

If you answered yes to one or more of these questions, you should seriously consider the possibility that you could be suffering from addiction. A professional evaluation may be necessary to be sure.

Alert

While online self-evaluation quizzes can be informative, interesting, and sometimes fun to take, they cannot take the place of a professional evaluation, diagnosis, and/or recommendation for treatment. Use them to increase awareness of a potential problem, then take action and seek professional mental health care for further help.

A physician or mental health professional who is knowledgeable and experienced in the treatment of addictions could work with you to confirm or deny that your substance use or compulsive behaviors are at the level of abuse or addiction. This may be done on an outpatient or inpatient basis, depending on the severity of symptoms. An addictionologist is the ideal professional to evaluate your situation. This is a physician who has completed additional specialized training in the evaluation and treatment of addictions. However, one may be difficult to find unless you live in a metropolitan area.

Recognizing Addictive Behaviors

If signs and symptoms of addiction are noticed in a loved one, don't shy away from asking questions and evaluating the situation. Addictions can be more than unpleasant—they can become downright destructive, and it is dangerous to ignore the early signs. Some signs of addiction are obvious and others are more subtle or may be interpreted as other disorders. For example, depression is a diagnosis all its own, but it may also be a symptom of addiction. Anxiety is another state that can be a symptom of addiction, as well as being a separate mental disorder. Those who are struggling with addictions may at first resent loved ones asking questions about their addictive behaviors. The addicted individual might be tempted to misinterpret the questions as his loved one intruding into his private business. If you are the one concerned about someone with addictions, don't let this put you off. Remember that distorted thinking is often a psychological effect of the addiction and an addicted loved one may not be thinking as clearly as usual. Once he has received effective treatment, he may very well be greatly appreciative of your efforts.

 Fact

Home drug-test kits are available. For example, *www.testmyteen.com* offers a urine drug-test kit that tests for ten of the most common illegal drugs: cocaine, amphetamine, marijuana, opiates, methamphetamine, barbiturates, benzodiazepines, oxycodone, Ecstacy, and narcotics.

If you are on the outside looking in and suspect that a friend or loved one might be involved in the use of an addictive substance or behavior, it is all right to express your concerns and try to help her identify the problem. Here are some ways you might approach your friend or loved one.

- First of all, reaffirm to your friend or loved one that you are talking with her and asking questions because you care for her welfare.
- Make noncritical observations about her change in habits (e.g., sleeping patterns, staying out all night, missing meals) and ask if these changes are related to substance use or compulsive behaviors.
- If teachers, coworkers, or bosses have been calling with complaints or concerns, let your loved one know, and ask for an explanation in a nonjudgmental manner. Let her know you are ready and willing to help with problems.
- In a loving but firm manner, confront lying and excuses as related to substance use or compulsive behaviors.
- Again, with a loving but firm approach, hold the addicted friend or loved one accountable for theft or breaking the law. Try to discover the facts of the situation if possible.

 Question

What kind of people are addicts?
Any type of person can struggle with addiction. Movie stars, doctors, lawyers, blue-collar workers, college students, and the homeless are all capable of becoming addicts. People of all racial and ethnic groups can develop addictions. The common denominator is body chemistry and how the brain reacts when a potentially addictive substance or behavior is introduced.

Always make it clear that you are asking questions because you care and want to help. You may be tempted to blame yourself for the addictions of your friend or loved one. Don't fall into this trap. You are not responsible. Neither is the addicted person responsible for the malfunctions in her brain that contribute to the addictive process. It is not helpful for the addicted person or those who care about her to avoid the signs and symptoms of addiction. This only delays identifying the problem and forming a plan to get help.

Effectively approaching a friend or loved one who may be struggling with addictions is not easy. It is common to fear anger or rejection. No one enjoys these difficult confrontations. However, it is important to remember that the purpose of the confrontation is to help the friend or loved one avoid difficult consequences, suffering, or even death. Approach him with a caring attitude. Make observations, ask questions that reflect a desire for information, and listen. Avoid blaming him or making accusations, as this approach is rarely effective. Make it clear that this is about helping him return to a healthier and more satisfying lifestyle.

Denial

Remember that denial is a hallmark symptom of addictions. It involves hiding the truth, refusing to talk about the problem, rationalizing, or minimizing the situation. Denial is a defensive measure on the part of the addicted person to avoid seeing the true nature of her problem and can significantly interfere with the identification process. This may be because the problem is too overwhelming or she fears failure. Even if an addict is forced to deal with a problem, such as filing for bankruptcy, denial says it has nothing to do with her compulsive spending or gambling. Losing one's job may be blamed on an unfair boss. Denial would lead a parent to blame a "vindictive" ex-spouse for his loss of visitation rights rather than admit that he drove the car drunk bringing the kids home from the last visit. Denial frequently comes across as making excuses—for example, "The other guys drink a lot more than I do," "Gambling is just entertainment, not an addiction—so what if I lost big this time, I can easily win it back plus more next week."

It is common for an addicted individual to have attempted quitting her addictive behaviors, and failed. She may have been trying to prove to herself that the problem behavior is not an addiction. This may have been done in secret, denying to others that there is any problem. However, the memory of the failure may lead her into further using the defensive measure of denial. She might try to convince herself that it didn't work in the past because she didn't *really* want to quit at that time.

Essential

Compulsory treatment programs are ineffective if the addicted person refuses to acknowledge his addiction. He will typically comply with treatment to avoid unpleasant consequences such as losing his driver's license, losing custody of his children, or having to go to jail, but he will resume his addiction as soon as the program has been completed.

An addicted person who is in denial will often vehemently deny that she has a problem. In fact, she asserts, she can quit any time she wants. She just hasn't had the desire to quit to this point. Be aware that denial may become more intense as the problems worsen. This is only a sign that the addicted person is in over her head and needs intensive help. However, if she is unwilling to face her use of denial, any treatment efforts will be ineffective. Acknowledgment of the addiction and the negative effects the addiction has on a person's life is necessary if true recovery is to take place. Further information about denial and how to overcome it will be discussed later.

CHAPTER 3

What Causes Addiction?

ADDICTIONS HAVE BEEN around for centuries. Over the years, many causative explanations have been proposed based on biological, genetic, social, and psychological factors. In spite of the many single-cause theories circulating in the field of addiction, it is more likely that a combination of factors results in addiction. This makes the understanding and treatment of addictions a complicated and ongoing process.

The Question of Willpower

In the early to mid 1800s, the addiction focus was on alcohol, and addiction was attributed to a person's weak character and spiritual disobedience. It was thought that if a person were closely following God, he would be able to make responsible choices related to addictions. Many institutions and organizations were developed during this time period to address these perceived moral and spiritual problems related to alcohol consumption. This causative theory still has its advocates even though there is now a multitude of evidence pointing to biological and genetic components that no one has the ability to control through willpower.

Dr. Benjamin Rush initially introduced what was a novel idea in 1784: addictions may have biological causes. At that time, Dr. Rush began to write about the consequences of chronic drunkenness and to expound his arguments that this was a biological disease that should be treated by physicians. By 1810, Dr. Rush was firmly advocating that alcoholism be seen as a biologically based disease and fought throughout the rest of his career to establish treatment programs to work with addicted individuals from a medical perspective. In 1825, Reverend Lyman Beecher wrote "Six Sermons on Intemperance" and warned people of the dangers of being addicted to distilled spirits. Dr. Samuel Woodward promoted creating inebriate asylums in 1830. A Home for the Fallen was opened in Boston in 1857. The movement to develop inebriate homes spread, and many alcoholic mutual aid societies were started.

 Fact

Dr. Magnus Huss, a Swedish physician, described chronic alcohol consumption as a disease, and in 1849 he named this disease Alcoholismus chronicus. This introduced the term alcoholism and further supported the notion that alcoholism is a disease rather than a spiritual or moral weakness.

Bill W. and Dr. Bob S. met for the first time in 1935. They recognized that on their own, they were powerless to conquer alcoholism, and in that same year founded Alcoholics Anonymous (A.A.), which continues to maintain an abstinent and spiritual basis for sobriety. *The Saturday Evening Post* wrote an article on Alcoholics Anonymous in 1941, and with this publication, A.A. began to spread around the country. It is now accepted that a lack of willpower or moral failure is not the cause of addictions and that willpower alone will not free a person from addictions. Social, medical, educational, spiritual, and psychiatric communities all have something to contribute in understanding the causes of addictions, and support from all quarters may be necessary for the addicted individual to achieve recovery.

Genetic Factors

Historically, things began to change in the United States in 1914, when the Harrison Anti-Narcotic Act brought opiates and cocaine under federal control. This placed physicians as the gatekeepers for legal access to these drugs. In 1935, a U.S. Public Health Prison Hospital opened in Lexington, Kentucky; a second facility opened in Fort Worth, Texas, in 1938. These two facilities were the sites of the first federal research programs in addiction treatment. Addiction research programs are now heavily involved in searching for genetic clues that will help explain the causes of addiction and provide effective solutions for treatment. This is encouraging news indeed if you are battling addictions.

Alert

Epidemiological studies have established that 40 percent to 60 percent of the risk for alcoholism is genetic. Similar rates of risk have been established for other drugs such as opiates and cocaine. It is therefore very important that a person with a family history of addictions avoid additional risk factors that encourage addictions.

It has been noted for a long time that addictions tend to run in families. In fact, children with alcoholic parents are four times more likely to become alcoholics than children of nonalcoholic parents. What exactly does that mean? Essentially, a genetic predisposition for addictions means that you metabolize drugs or alcohol differently than individuals without genetic tendencies. This is similar to the way cardiovascular diseases, high blood pressure, diabetes, and other diseases run in families. Researchers have identified several large chromosomal regions that are likely involved in addictions. As you can imagine, the addictive process is quite complicated, and this certainly presents a significant problem in identifying specific genes related to addictions. In spite of the complexities, forward strides are being made. Recent research has suggested that chromosome 17 is involved in addictions. It has been proposed that chromosome 6 may be involved in opiate addiction. It seems that the AGS3 gene in an area of the forebrain called the nucleus accumbens is likely involved in heroin addiction.

 Fact

Because of the moral and ethical problems of conducting genetic research in humans, laboratory mice and rats are bred to respond to drugs of abuse. The mechanism of genetic factors in addictions are then studied in the animal models before applying the research to humans.

The truth is, any single gene may produce a very small effect on the body's ability to develop an addiction and therefore be difficult to detect. More and more it seems that there are many genes associated with addictions.

Biological Factors

Biological changes in the brain can also lead to addictions. The dopamine pleasure circuit is not the only part of the brain involved in addictions. The prefrontal cortex located in the frontal lobe of the brain can also be affected. The prefrontal cortex is involved in our ability to make logical, rational, and appropriate decisions. In a non-addicted individual, the dopamine pleasure circuit is in balance with our prefrontal cortex. If a person experiences the euphoric feeling of cocaine, the dopamine pleasure circuit would be in favor of pursuing that activity. The prefrontal cortex would balance this urge by helping the person think through the subsequent consequences of using an illegal drug. However, when the usual balance between the dopamine pleasure circuit and the prefrontal cortex is disrupted by the introduction of excessive amounts of dopamine, the potential to develop an addiction has occurred. The dopamine pleasure circuit wins out and the addicted individual experiences a decreased capacity to make healthy choices related to addictive substances or behaviors.

What often happens is that a person will use a potentially addictive substance out of curiosity or a desire to experiment. Once the dopamine pleasure circuit is activated by the substance of abuse, the body's natural reward/pleasure pathways are disrupted. Because drugs of abuse are often capable of releasing two to ten times more dopamine than the body's natural system, a more powerful reward system is artificially developed. The person's brain system becomes altered and there is a hunger for more of the addictive substance to obtain feelings of pleasure. An addiction is born.

 Question

Why do adolescents seem particularly prone to developing addictions?
The prefrontal cortex is the last part of the brain to develop, and so the immature brains of children and adolescents are less able to manage both the decisions involved in starting addictions and the ability to chemically handle addictions. Therefore, once an addictive substance is introduced into the adolescent's brain, the dopamine pleasure circuit tends to dominate decision-making.

Environmental Factors

A prime environmental factor in causing addictions is the availability of the substance or supplies needed to engage in the addictive behavior. Addictive substances can be obtained in schools, on the streets of the community, or in the home. At one time, the focus was on drug dealers based in the criminal world as suppliers of illicit substances. They were seen as the core of the drug threat to the community in terms of availability. It is now known that a supplier could be a criminal drug dealer, but could also be a neighbor, a child's friends at school, a business associate, or even a parent.

Availability doesn't always involve buying and selling. One group of addictive substances that is readily available in everyone's home, in the classroom, or in the workplace has already been mentioned: inhalants. Marijuana, another commonly used addictive substance, can be grown in one's own backyard.

Essential

The public health model of addictions involves three causative factors. One factor is the addictive substance itself. Another factor is the person with the potential to become addicted. A final factor is the environment, which includes availability of the addictive substance. In this causative model, all three factors are necessary for addiction to occur.

Methamphetamines are another addictive substance that can be manufactured in a person's home with readily available chemicals and common cold remedies. Laws attempting to limit the manufacture of methamphetamines are being passed in many states. Encouraging or requiring retailers to identify individuals who purchase large quantities of products that could be used to manufacture methamphetamines is one example. Common cold remedies are now being stocked behind retail counters rather than on shelves where it's harder to monitor their purchase.

A lack of community involvement or a lack of attachment to a community is another environmental element that seems to play a part in promoting addictions. Participating in satisfying community relationships and contributing to worthwhile community projects are protective measures against addictions. Communities that are lacking in opportunities for people to socially connect in satisfying ways may become significant factors in the development of addictions. Communities with high crime rates statistically have higher rates of addiction. This makes sense when one thinks of the multiple crimes committed in connection with addictions. Knowing that another person cares is a powerful factor in preventing addictions or in encouraging someone already addicted to seek help.

Family Relations and Learned Behavior

Family influences on the development of addictions can be very powerful. There are the genetic influences that have already been discussed. Families can also influence the development of addictions by example. A child who watches his parents or other adult relatives using substances or engaging in other addictive behaviors gets the message that this is acceptable. It is typical childhood behavior to want to emulate significant adults in one's life. The child is often looking for adult approval when she copies the adult's behavior. In families where addictions are openly practiced, young people may be purposely introduced to and included in the addiction. This may be seen as an acceptable custom common to the family culture. In families where physical, verbal, emotional, and sexual abuse may be present, it is not uncommon for a person to begin using addictive substances at an early age to escape the emotional pain. Once a person discovers that he can numb the emotional pain with addictive substances or behaviors, he typically continues this practice on into adulthood.

 Alert

It is now confirmed that childhood trauma has the capability of altering the brain. Changes in the brain that occur as the result of childhood trauma, such as physical or sexual abuse, can cause a person to be more susceptible to addictions.

Social learning theory has contributed significantly to understanding the social causes of addiction. Social learning theory is a psychological concept that attempts to explain through a set of observations how a person learns behaviors through social interactions. There are four stages in social learning theory that may explain a potential addict's behavior, the first of which involves attention. The potential addict makes a conscious choice to watch others engaging in addictive behaviors. Memory is the second stage, with the individual recalling what he has observed. The third stage is imitation. In this stage, the individual repeats the behaviors that he has observed. Motivation is the fourth stage. If the addictive behavior is to be imitated and carried out, there must be some internal motivation for the individual to do so. How does this learning theory apply to the development of addictions? The addictive behavior of a friend, family member, peer, or other admired individual gets one's attention. An addict may remember watching addictive behaviors in those people he looked up to or admired. At some point, he may have made a choice to try the addictive substance or behavior that he observed. The internal motivation he may have felt to continue using the addictive substance or behavior may have been the approval of the person being imitated, or the numbing of emotional pain, or the stimulation of the pleasure pathway in his brain. All of this may have happened at either a conscious or an unconscious level.

Essential

Once an individual becomes addicted to substances or behaviors, family attention often shifts from family issues to the addict. It is common for the addicted person to be blamed for family problems at this point. The stress of unresolved family problems can contribute to the development and perpetuation of addictions.

Responses such as stimulation of the pleasure pathway serve as positive reinforcement, which keeps the addictive behavior going. Positive reinforcement in this case is when one experiences good feelings such as mellowness, euphoria, relaxation, or a "high" after use of a substance or addictive behavior. Positive reinforcement also occurs when a person experiences acceptance from others who use addictive substances or behaviors.

Psychological Factors

Remember that it is common for a person to self-medicate to cope with her problems. If someone seeks to find relief from emotional difficulties through substances or compulsive behaviors, she may develop addictions. This is a popular perspective on the cause of addictions. Addictive substances and/or behaviors may be used to relieve one's stress, to improve one's mood, and to relieve one's emotional pain and discomfort. It is currently well known that addictions frequently go hand in hand with mood disorders and other psychological problems. Mental health problems that are frequently seen coexisting with addictions can include anxiety disorders, bipolar disorder, depression, obsessive-compulsive disorder, and personality disorders.

 Question

What is a dual diagnosis?
When addictions to alcohol, substances, and/or compulsive behaviors are diagnosed simultaneously with a mental disorder or psychiatric problem, this is known as a dual diagnosis. According to the 2002 National Survey on Drug Use and Health, 17.5 million adults were diagnosed with a serious mental illness in the United States. Four million of those adults met the criteria for both a serious mental illness and addiction.

Certain psychiatric disorders may particularly increase your risk for addictions. Those disorders associated with an increased risk for addictions include attention deficit hyperactivity disorder (ADHD), post-traumatic stress disorder (PTSD), antisocial personality disorder, bipolar disorder, schizophrenia, and major depressive disorder. If someone has both a psychiatric disorder and an addiction, both must be effectively treated if that person is to successfully recover from both. As with addictions, psychiatric disorders also have multiple causes, including genetics, environmental factors, physiological components, and social influences. If this is the situation, it will be important to understand and appreciate the complexity of treating both psychiatric disorders and addictions simultaneously. At times, the symptoms of addiction can mask the symptoms of a psychiatric disorder, and vice versa. A professional with specialized training is necessary in order to treat a dually diagnosed person effectively. This is not something that a person can manage successfully on her own or even with the help of friends and family.

 Fact

> Two common myths about addictions are that addicts are bad, crazy, or stupid, and that, since addictions are often treated with behavioral approaches, the addictions must be caused by behavioral problems. Myths fail to take into account the fact that addictions are now known to involve changes in the brain and many other causative factors.

Another psychological theory to be aware of is that illogical thinking may lead to addictions. This explanation assumes that an addict is controlled by distorted and unreasonable thoughts. An example of a distorted thought would be when a person who was addicted to gambling believed that she could win every time she entered a casino. If someone were addicted to alcohol, it would be an unreasonable thought to expect other family members to go without adequate food and clothing so the addict could afford to buy his substance. The foundation of treatment based on this theory is that a person's thinking needs to be challenged for accuracy.

Negative self-talk also puts a susceptible individual at risk for addictions. Examples of negative self-talk include catastrophizing, minimizing, blaming, perfectionism, magnifying, and so forth. Catastrophizing is always expecting the worst to happen. Minimizing makes less of something than what is actually there. Perfectionists tend to set impossible standards for themselves and others. If someone magnifies an event, she makes more of it than is warranted by the situation. Negative self-talk can provide rationalizations for substance use and addictive behaviors. The treatment for negative self-talk is to rewrite the message to reflect an accurate perspective.

An Addictive Personality

Many have wondered if there is an "addictive personality." Whether an addictive personality exists has been debated for years. If there is such a thing, does an addictive personality cause addictive behavior or is it the result of addiction? After many years of research, the theory of an addictive personality is not supported by experts; nevertheless, the notion of an addictive personality persists. Certain personality traits continue to be associated with addicted individuals. These associations have kept alive the idea that personality may be a causative factor in addictions. Examples of these personality traits include:

- Impulsiveness and problems delaying gratification
- Enjoyment of risk-taking and seeking sensationalism
- Pride about being a nonconformist and devaluation of typical achievement goals put forth in society
- Social isolation and problems connecting with others in meaningful relationships
- Consistent feelings of anxiety and problems managing stress on a regular basis
- Demonstration of antisocial traits such as not caring how one's actions affect others
- Compulsive behaviors

- Manipulation and self-centeredness
- Dependency on others

Again, whether these characteristics compose an "addictive personality" or whether there are other explanations that account for these qualities has yet to be definitively determined.

Alert

> The complexity of factors that combine to cause addictions are reflected in a formula described by Dennis C. Daley in his book, *Addiction and Mood Disorders*. His formula is: Biology + Psychology + Family Influences + Social Influences + Alcohol/Drugs = Addiction.

A valid observation regarding the traits of an "addictive personality" is that they could also be symptoms of various psychiatric disorders. Impulsiveness is a hallmark feature of ADHD; obsessive-compulsive disorder and generalized anxiety disorder also include some of these qualities. One cannot exclude the personality disorders, either. Antisocial personality disorder with attention focused on meeting one's own needs or wants regardless of the effect on others has long been associated with addictive behaviors as well. Individuals with borderline personality disorder are commonly known to seek out the sensational and take excessive risks. Although an addicted person may exhibit a unique personality profile, there may also be underlying psychiatric problems that are compatible with the use of addictive substances and behaviors.

CHAPTER 4

Cultural Lures and Addiction

THE NEWS AND advertising media give a lot of coverage to addiction—the lure of addictive substances and behaviors as well as the consequences of becoming addicted. Certainly it's not all bad news. Advancements in knowledge and treatment techniques is excellent news for anyone who struggles with addictions. But advertising and celebrity news, for instance, put a susceptible person in a position of daily having to make choices related to addictions. That can be a lot of pressure. The associations between glamour, entertainment, and addictions are present and unavoidable.

Advertising Is Everywhere

It's true; advertising is everywhere and a person can't open his eyes or ears in the morning without being exposed to it in some form. Morning, noon, and night, the food addict is faced with commercials that may trigger her desire to eat foods that will lead to a binge. Beer commercials are present with almost every sporting event. Movies, television, billboards, radio, Internet, newspapers, magazines, and shopping malls are all filled with advertisements. Advertising is an accepted way of life in American culture as a means of selling goods and services. Even if particular addictive substances or behaviors are not directly advertised, people in commercials, advertisements, and public entertainment may be depicted using addictive substances and engaging in addictive behaviors in ways that appear very attractive. It is not hard to sell addictions. Just remember the pleasure pathway and the hedonic highway. Addictions often feel good in the moment, and it can be challenging at times to remember the negative consequences that are inevitable down the road. Does this mean that earplugs and blinders should be part of one's daily wardrobe when leaving the house? No, but it does mean that awareness of the agenda of advertisers must be constantly present.

 Fact

According to *MedPage Today* (August 2007), alcohol ads accounted for 43.9 percent of all magazine advertising in 2005. Alcohol advertising on television programs frequently watched by youth increased 41 percent between 2001 and 2005. These statistics clearly demonstrate the pervasive level of exposure to the public of at least one potentially addictive substance.

Why Advertising Is So Effective

Advertising is effective because it is designed to appeal to one's pleasure senses. Advertising is also designed to make a person believe that life can be easy, fun, and irresponsible without consequences. It leads one to believe that the pleasure of the moment is all that counts. Advertising definitely takes advantage of the altered prefrontal cortex in addicted individuals. It may be the key that unlocks the gate leading to the pleasure pathway through presenting triggers to susceptible individuals.

Take casinos, for example. Casinos advertise free food, exciting and entertaining shows with celebrities, and a chance to win easy money. Many high schools and colleges have "Vegas" night with blackjack tables, crap tables, and poker for students to indulge in for entertainment. If schools sponsor this type of activity, it must be safe and fun, right? Think about this. Eighteen-year-old young adults become eligible for credit cards simultaneously with being allowed into casinos. Does that mean all eighteen-year-olds are going to gamble their lives away? Of course not. But the young adult who is tempted to gamble can easily get in over his head in debt before he knows it and develop an addiction with lifelong consequences.

This doesn't just happen at casinos, either. Shopping malls have amazing displays designed for the young consumer. Discounts are given in many department stores if one uses a credit card instead of cash. This can be a huge temptation for someone who just received that first credit card in the mail and can't wait to try it out. If a person has a tendency toward addictive spending, this may be the entry into a long battle with shopping addiction. Availability doesn't automatically lead to addictions, but it does make it easier to get started.

The Curiosity Factor

A child or an adolescent in particular may have great curiosity about the things he encounters in the world. Curiosity is normal and to be encouraged in many areas. Drugs and alcohol are not areas where curiosity should be indulged. R-rated movies are one activity that can be tantalizing to many children and adolescents. These movies are associated with adult material and kids may mistakenly feel "adult" watching them and emulating the behaviors seen in these movies.

 Question

How do R-rated movies affect children?
KidsHealth reported on a study conducted between 2002 and 2003 with 2,606 nine- to twelve-year-old children. Results indicated that 55 percent of the children watched R-rated movies, with only one-third of those children always watching the movies with parents. Children who never watched R-rated movies were at least 40 percent less likely to engage in smoking and drinking.

Adult movies often provide a showcase for many potentially addictive substances and behaviors presented as entertainment. This is a dangerous message, particularly for young people in their teen years whose frontal lobes aren't as developed and who may not be able to readily think through the long-term implications of what they're seeing. Parental supervision is absolutely necessary in the selection of children's and teens' entertainment. When it comes to movies, it may be wise to limit the movies watched by children and teens to those rated PG-13 and below, in spite of the child's curiosity and desire to be more "adult." This is equally true for video, arcade, and computer games. Games are now also rated for good reason. Sexually explicit material and drug-related material is rampant in many games. Watching models of substance use and compulsive behaviors as depicted in movies, television, video games, and music videos has an effect even more powerful than direct advertisements. Social learning through modeling admired examples is very powerful, particularly for young people, who may be more impressionable.

 Fact

On July 26, 2007, the Center on Media and Child Health reported that Disney would no longer allow presentations of smoking in Disney movies and would discourage smoking in Touchstone and Miramax movies, which Disney also owns. This was in response to a study that found smoking present in 64 percent of Disney's youth-rated movies between 1999 and 2006.

Many men have reported that a pornography addiction was born out of curiosity. They frequently describe having found pornographic magazines, books, or movies in their father's closet or in a trash can somewhere during childhood or adolescence. Peers may have brought some of this forbidden material to school and boys may have felt thrilled to be included in looking at pornographic material on the playground at recess. Curiosity is a very powerful force that often feels irresistible. Although men are certainly not alone in their curiosity about pornography, a much greater percentage of men than women are drawn into this activity.

Why is exposure to potentially addictive substances and behaviors such a big deal? Recall the discussion of the dopamine reward circuit. Once a pleasurable experience is associated with an addictive substance or behavior, that experience is recorded in memories. The addictive substance or behavior establishes connections between the addictive experience and the circumstances under which it occurred through changes in the brain. Technically speaking, the nucleus accumbens sends signals to the amygdala and hippocampus. The amygdala and hippocampus then record and consolidate memories that have evoked strong feelings. Each time an addicted individual is exposed to the circumstances that have been connected with pleasant memories of addiction, she will be tempted to engage in the addiction again.

Alert

Pleasurable experiences that are set in motion by addictive substances or behaviors trigger biological processes resulting in overloading the nucleus accumbens with dopamine. Thus, addictions become a shortcut to pleasurable sensations and natural rewards are no longer satisfying.

Peer Pressure and Social Expectations

The pressure to engage in the use of potentially addicting substances and behaviors is hard to avoid. Children and adolescents are not the only ones who experience social pressure. Adults also have to deal with temptations that might lead to addiction. Weddings, bar mitzvahs, job-promotion parties, New Year's Eve celebrations, and even the innocuous birthday party can feel like land mines that have to be negotiated! A food addict may not get much understanding when he refuses a piece of his own birthday cake. How can a groom struggling with alcoholism say no to the traditional champagne toast at his wedding? Saying no to these things is possible, but often comes with disapproving glances and comments from people whose approval and opinions matter. Individuals who do not struggle with addictions may have a hard time understanding why total abstinence may be necessary for recovery.

 Question

What is an "alcopop"?
An alcopop is a premixed fruity drink made with alcoholic beverages and fruit juices. "Hard" lemonade and wine coolers made with various fruit juices are examples of alcopops. A person can easily deceive herself into thinking these drinks are nonaddictive because of the juice ingredient, and because they are often packaged to look like soda pop or other nonalcoholic drinks. However, if enough is consumed, they can still be addictive.

Social pressure or peer pressure appeals to one's desire to fit in with others, to experience acceptance and approval. There is nothing inherently wrong with this. Human beings are primarily social creatures and are born with a drive to connect with other human beings. It is very satisfying to know that one is pleasing and acceptable to significant individuals in one's life. However, when that desire for social belonging is paired with pressure to use addictive substances or engage in addictive behaviors, things get tough.

Influence by Celebrities

It is interesting to note how much influence celebrities have in our culture. People who have no personal connection or relationship to the "man on the street," so to speak, have input into one's hairstyle, clothing, mannerisms, and even the cologne one wears. Celebrities can also influence what a person does for entertainment, what food one eats, and one's beverage of choice. In times past, this level of influence primarily came from one's parents, extended family, teachers, and neighbors. Mass media has changed everything.

Essential

Pseudo-relationships can develop between celebrities and their fans. There may be an illusion of friendship or even a feeling of intimacy that is one-sided. Celebrities have a sphere of influence through the media whereby they can model and encourage by example the use of addictive substances or ways to live healthy lives.

Watching celebrities engaging in substance use or addictive behaviors in movies or music videos can lead to learned behavior by modeling. Remember that modeling through social learning can have a very significant environmental effect on developing addictions. Young people may idolize celebrities who glorify substance use in movies, music, and other media forms. It can be very confusing to a young person who idolizes a celebrity and desires to copy the celebrity's behavior to see a very unappealing "mug shot" in the news when that celebrity is arrested for drunk driving or substance abuse. This has happened many times in recent years, with some celebrities earning jail time for their activities. Of course, celebrities can also have a positive effect on their fans by modeling the resistance of potentially addictive substances or behaviors. Celebrities can also model changed lives if they have been addicted and are seen living out responsible recovery.

While movies, television programs, and music videos may find a more receptive audience in young people, adults are not immune. Adults and children may also be influenced by celebrities from other areas of interest. Take sports, for example. Even though professional athletes are regularly monitored for illicit substance use, sports figures are continually seen highlighted in the news for substance abuse, gambling addiction, and other addictions. Sports figures are frequently featured in commercials and advertisements for alcohol. There has been considerable controversy in recent years over the illegal use of steroids by athletes. This isn't to say that there aren't many professional athletes who take their role of being positive examples very seriously. They are to be commended and they can have a powerful positive influence on their fans.

Ethnic and Cultural Differences

Just as the development of addictions may be influenced by celebrities, advertising, and the media in the United States, it may also be influenced by culture and ethnicity. Cultural beliefs and practices do indeed affect how individuals view the use of addictive substances and compulsive behaviors. Some groups still view addictions as moral weaknesses. These groups do not accept the disease model of addiction and expect individuals to manage their addictions through willpower and choices. If an addicted individual is unable to gain control of his addictive process in this manner, he may find himself excluded from the social group. In addition to the problem of addiction, the addicted individual may also suffer the emotional trauma of social ostracism.

Problems with acculturation may be a significant influence on addictions in the lives of individuals from different ethnic groups. The United States is still a melting pot, consisting of people from a variety of cultural groups originating from all over the world. For instance, there are some drugs, such as peyote or cannabis, that are commonly used as parts of religious ceremonies in certain cultures. Some of these practices may be illegal in the United States. Changes in long-established cultural traditions are required in order to comply with the law.

Alcohol runs the gamut in different cultures. It may be forbidden for some and encouraged in others. In some cultures, drug and alcohol problems may be seen as due to destiny or fate, or they may be attributed to supernatural causes. Family ties are very important in certain ethnic groups, and an individual struggling with addictions could be considered an embarrassment to the family. These are some of the barriers that may need to be overcome for an individual to receive effective treatment. Sometimes the pressure of trying to fit into a different culture may itself lead to the development of addictions in order to cope. Social conditions such as acculturation, extreme poverty, and discrimination are primary factors affecting the use of alcohol and substances among different cultural and ethnic groups.

 Alert

Different cultural and ethnic groups have varying perspectives on addictions that may have developed over hundreds of years. It is very important that these perspectives be respected and taken into consideration when developing a treatment plan to help addicted individuals.

Dealing with External Pressures

The greatest safeguards against external pressures to become involved with addictive substances or behaviors are knowledge and awareness. Education on the dangers of addiction can also help you identify triggers. A trigger is a stimulus that at one time had no significant effect on an individual. Repeated associations between that previously insignificant stimulus and addictive substances or behaviors subsequently leads to cravings whenever that stimulus is encountered. For example, a football game in and of itself, has no relationship to addictions. However, when an individual watches beer commercials that use football players as spokesmen and then consistently drinks beer every time he watches a football game, a connection develops. He can no longer watch a football game without feeling the urge to drink a beer.

It is extremely important to be aware of external pressures to succumb to addictions and how those pressures work as enticements. Surrounding oneself with positive influences and healthy examples is of inestimable benefit. Healthy self-esteem and self-confidence are two of the best insulators against addictions. Be honest about your weaknesses as well as your strengths. Thus, when one feels tempted to manage weaknesses with addictions, the temptation can be recognized and one can turn to more beneficial ways to deal with problems.

As a parent, you can provide your young or adolescent children with activities they can excel at and thus build their self-esteem in a positive way. Help your children objectively evaluate the music, movies, television programs, and video games they watch. When your child's favorite sports star is exposed with addiction problems, help him view that person with compassion while at the same time guiding him to understand the potential consequences of addictive behaviors.

Seeking Help

Just as cultural and advertising influences can have a negative impact on addictions, they can also turn an individual around in a positive direction. Many people in the United States have been encouraged to seek treatment because of former first lady Betty Ford, who went public with her alcoholism. Her well-known struggles and recovery became an example of courage. The Betty Ford Center is now a model for treatment centers around the country. Facing the stigma of addictions is a first step for an individual to take in seeking help. Find an outpatient professional, a treatment program, or a support group that meets your particular needs. Different addictions will require different treatment approaches. Don't hesitate to interview professionals before engaging their services. Make certain they are culturally sensitive and knowledgeable, clinically competent, and adequately available. Acknowledge your own courage in seeking help, honor your efforts, and celebrate your progress.

CHAPTER 5

Alcohol Addiction

ALCOHOL ADDICTION, ALCOHOLISM, and alcohol dependence are equivalent terms that refer to a physiological dependence on alcohol characterized by the development of tolerance and withdrawal symptoms. Alcohol is a multifaceted substance. Initially, it may act as a stimulant or have uninhibiting effects. However, continued drinking leads to its primary effect, that of a depressant. It has a negative effect on moods, behavior, and physiology.

What Is Alcoholism?

Alcoholism is a chronic and progressive disease that has a predictable course, recognizable symptoms, and genetic and environmental foundations. It includes the characteristics of craving, development of tolerance, and withdrawal symptoms when attempting to cut down or stop drinking. Alcoholism drives one to continued drinking in spite of adverse health and social consequences.

The Brain

The real story of alcoholism begins in the brain. Alcohol interferes with the brain's neurotransmitters. GABA (gamma-aminobutyric acid) is an inhibitory neurotransmitter and promotes feelings of calmness in the brain. NMDA (N-methyl-D-aspartate) is a glutamate that acts as an excitatory neurotransmitter, promoting activity and growth in the brain. In healthy brain functioning, these two neurotransmitters, as with other brain chemicals, are in balance. However, alcohol shuts down NMDA and allows GABA to take over. When this occurs, a person experiences slowed communication, reduced motor coordination, slurred speech, and eventually blackouts. NMDA is necessary for learning and memory, so when NMDA functioning is abnormal, learning and memory suffer. Furthermore, alcohol interferes with the supply of tryptophan, an amino acid that promotes the release of serotonin. Serotonin is another neurotransmitter involved in mood regulation. A decrease in the levels or functioning of serotonin leads to depression and/or anxiety. Alcohol addiction has also been associated with low levels of MAO (monoamine oxidase) and CREB (cyclic AMP response element-binding protein). MAO is an enzyme that breaks down certain neurotransmitters such as serotonin, norepinephrine, and dopamine. Decreased amounts of MAO are associated with impulsivity, short attention span, pleasure-seeking, and a low pain threshold. CREB is associated with long-term memory formation, and a lowered level has also been associated with anxiety in alcoholics.

Alert

Unquestionably, alcohol poses a significant problem in this country. About half of all American adults drink alcohol. Statistics show that approximately one-third of adults have had alcohol-related problems. Approximately 10 percent of women and 20 percent of men abuse alcohol, while 5 percent of women and 10 percent of men have the disease of alcoholism.

Alcohol has harmful effects on the medulla, the part of the brain that controls basic survival functions. Therefore, alcohol can affect the brain's ability to moderate breathing and heart rate. As if that were not enough, alcohol addiction can also lead to premature aging, especially for someone over forty years of age. In studies of the brains of alcoholic men, it has been found that there is decreased blood flow to the frontal lobe of the brain, an area associated with memory, creativity, and problem-solving. The nerve membranes are affected, which can lead to structural changes and damage to this part of the brain. An individual who has consumed alcohol heavily for thirty to forty years may have a brain that weighs as much as 105 grams less than an individual who drank lightly or not at all.

 Fact

Alcohol kills brain cells, especially those in the left hemisphere of the brain. The left hemisphere is associated with the development of language and the ability to use logic. An alcoholic will lose approximately 60,000 more brain cells per day than a person who drinks lightly or not at all.

Other Physiological Effects of Alcohol

As significant as the effects of alcohol are on the brain, the rest of the body is not left out. The liver is the primary site where alcohol is metabolized or broken down. When the liver becomes overburdened by having to deal with too much alcohol, it becomes damaged. Three liver disorders attributed to alcohol are fatty liver (an excessive accumulation of fats, particularly triglycerides, in the liver), alcoholic hepatitis (a combination of fatty liver, inflammation of the liver, and the death of healthy liver cells), and alcoholic cirrhosis (the replacement of healthy liver tissue with nonfunctioning scar tissue). There is no known cure for cirrhosis and it can lead to liver cancer or complete liver failure, both of which can be fatal.

As with all foods and drinks, alcohol passes through the digestive system—the esophagus, stomach, and pancreas. In the esophagus, alcohol can cause reflux, leading to esophagitis, an inflammation of the esophagus. Complications of alcohol addiction, such as increased blood pressure in the primary vein carrying blood from the intestines to the liver, can also lead to the development of swollen and distended veins in the esophagus. If those veins rupture, death may result. Gastritis, an inflammation of the stomach lining, is also common in alcoholics. It can prevent the effective absorption of food and medicines, which obviously leads to additional problems. Untreated, gastritis can also be fatal. Alcohol can inhibit the body's healing process; in the stomach, this can lead to an aggravation of stomach ulcers. Alcohol can start an ulcer through the stimulation of excessive production of gastric juices. The pancreas produces enzymes required for digestion and insulin, which controls blood sugar levels. Pancreatitis, or inflammation of the pancreas, is also common in alcoholics and may be fatal. Heavy drinking can also lead to hypertension (high blood pressure), cardiomyopathy (disease of the heart muscle), and stroke. Binge drinking in particular can cause irregular heartbeats, palpitations, and even sudden death.

 Question

What is alcohol poisoning?
Alcohol poisoning can occur when a large amount of alcohol is consumed over a short amount of time. The liver is overwhelmed and cannot metabolize the alcohol as fast as it is consumed. In alcohol poisoning, the blood alcohol level may be as high as 0.4—five times the legal limit for driving. Alcohol poisoning can be fatal.

Lesser-known effects of alcohol on the body include contributing to osteoporosis in the bones. Gout, a painful swelling of joints, is worsened by alcohol and is quite difficult to treat. Alcohol can cause diseases in the muscles and skin as well. Because of its effects on the immune system, alcohol has played a significant part in the development of tuberculosis, pneumonia, and infections associated with AIDS. Sexual problems due to alcohol include temporary impotence in men and a failure to ovulate in women. Heavy alcohol use is connected with many types of cancer: mouth, larynx, pharynx, esophagus, liver, stomach, colon, rectal, and breast.

Mental Health Problems

With all the effects on the brain that have been presented, it is no surprise that alcohol also leads to many mental health problems. Primary among these problems are depression and anxiety, related to alcohol's tendency to interfere with neurotransmitters that affect moods. A very serious brain disorder common in long-term alcoholics is called Wernicke's encephalopathy. It is caused by a deficiency in Vitamin B_1 (thiamine). As alcoholism progresses, the alcoholic's craving for his substance is greater than his desire for food. Malnutrition results, which is where vitamin deficiencies come in to play. Symptoms experienced with Wernicke's encephalopathy include confusion, drowsiness, poor balance, double vision, and abnormal eye movements.

Essential

Medications can intensify the effects of alcohol. This is especially true for medications that slow down the central nervous system, such as sleeping medications, antihistamines, antidepressants, anti-anxiety medications, and some pain medications. Medications used to treat diabetes and heart disease can also have a dangerous interaction effect with alcohol. Check specifics with a physician and be careful!

If untreated, Wernicke's encephalopathy can progress to Korsakoff's syndrome. This is a very serious illness with the key component being memory loss. A person with this disorder can neither recall old events nor form new memories.

Genetics

Many of the research studies done to determine if there is a genetic link to alcoholism involve comparisons between biological siblings, twins, and adopted family members. Studies are consistently finding that biological children of alcoholic parents are two to three times more likely to become alcoholics than biological children of nonalcoholic parents. A study of identical male twins with alcoholic parents found they had 50 to 200 percent greater likelihood of developing alcoholism than fraternal male twins. Identical twins have the same genetic makeup. Research in this area is really just getting started. Thus far, it seems there may be a genetic link between alcoholism and chromosomes 1 and 4. The dopamine D2 receptor gene (DRD2) and a gene called ankyrin repeat and kinase domain containing 1 (ANKK1) have also been associated with alcoholism.

 Alert

> It has been estimated that alcoholism can reduce a person's life expectancy by ten years. Diseases such as cancers, heart disease, liver disease, and so forth take their toll. Additionally, there are deaths due to suicides and traffic fatalities related to alcohol.

Although this information on genetics is still being confirmed, it is clear that genetics do play a part in alcoholism. At the same time, it is important to remember that just because a person may have the genetic tendency to become an alcoholic doesn't mean he or she will automatically become one. Many other factors also contribute to the development of alcoholism.

The "Social Drinker"

Can an individual be a social drinker? The answer is yes, with exceptions. Social drinking is defined as light drinking within the context of a social situation such as meals, parties, dates, or recreational events with friends. Social drinking is not drinking to the point of drunkenness and it is not binge drinking. The primary characteristics of social drinking include:

- Enjoying alcohol in a social context but not being preoccupied with drinking
- Going for long periods without alcohol and not experiencing anxiety
- Genuinely being able to stop drinking at any time
- Being in total control of how much alcohol is consumed
- Not experiencing the adverse consequences of alcohol, such as problems with law enforcement

Two drinks per day for men and one drink per day for women and older people consumed in a safe, legal, and responsible manner is considered social drinking. Blood alcohol concentration (BAC) is the amount of alcohol in the blood and is measured in milligrams of alcohol per 100 milliliters of blood, or milligrams percent. The BAC range of social drinking is .00 to .05 percent. This means that 5/100 of 1 percent of the total blood content is alcohol. Within this range, one might feel slightly relaxed or a little lightheaded. There may be a loosening of inhibitions or even a mild sense of euphoria. A person might find himself beginning to talk more rapidly and behaviors may become slightly exaggerated.

 Question

How much is considered to be one drink?
The amount in one drink may actually be far less than you imagined. A person in denial may gradually begin to increase what she would describe as "a" drink. But the fact is that one drink is one twelve-ounce bottle of beer or wine cooler, one five-ounce glass of wine, or one and a half ounces of eighty-proof distilled liquor.

Remember that social drinking is just that—social. It is drinking within a relational context. This means that it is important to carefully choose your drinking friends. Young people in particular are strongly influenced to adapt to the drinking patterns of their friends.

The amount of alcohol consumed in social situations is often strongly determined by how much others in the group are drinking. Most individuals experience few adverse side effects if they remain within the realm of genuine light social drinking. Heavier social drinking, which is as little as three drinks a day, can actually lead to brain damage. Heavy social drinkers generally function well at home and at their jobs. Therefore, they appear to have no problems with this level of drinking. However, research has demonstrated that heavy social drinkers may experience a loss of brain cells and brain metabolite changes similar to alcoholics, but less severe. A heavy social drinker may have problems with abstract concepts, memory, and thinking ahead about future consequences.

Finally, there are certain situations in which even social drinking should be avoided. It is never considered safe for a woman who is pregnant or attempting to become pregnant to drink any amount of alcohol. Some medical conditions, such as cirrhosis of the liver, may be worsened by drinking alcohol. Also, one must be careful when taking certain medications, including over-the-counter medications, that there are no harmful interactions with alcohol. Ask a physician or pharmacist if you have any doubt. Alcohol is not recommended for recovering alcoholics or individuals suffering from psychological disorders. And of course, it is never a smart move to mix alcohol with driving.

The Effects of Alcohol on Moods

Alcohol has long been used as a method of relaxation. Having a drink to unwind from a stressful day is a common practice in our culture. Anxiety seems to dissolve, at least temporarily, with a glass of wine or a beer. In small amounts, this may be effective. For a person susceptible to alcohol addiction or who has a mood disorder, it may not be wise. It has long been noted that alcohol affects moods and moods have influenced the use of alcohol. Mood disorders include anxiety, depression, and bipolar disorder. When alcoholism and mood disorders coexist, this is referred to as a dual disorder. However, it is important to recognize that just because a person is addicted to alcohol doesn't automatically mean she also suffers from a mental illness. Alcohol can cause mood disorder symptoms to worsen, and it can interfere with medications used to treat mood disorders, thus prolonging recovery.

Alert

Remember that alcohol has the ability to impair judgment. A person with a major depressive disorder who also drinks alcohol excessively is at risk for suicide. In fact, according to Dr. Esther Gwinnell and Christine Adamec in their book, *The Encyclopedia of Addictions and Addictive Behaviors*, the risk of suicide for both men and women has been reported to be thirty times higher in alcoholics than among the general population.

The manic symptoms of bipolar disorder can be triggered by alcohol use; on the other hand, a person might self-medicate the manic symptoms with the depressant effects of alcohol. A significant danger to be aware of is that alcohol can mask psychiatric disorders, particularly mood disorders. Depression, for example, may be mistakenly thought to be due to the effects of alcohol. While it is true that alcohol is a depressant, only a skilled professional may be able to determine whether there is also an underlying major depressive disorder. The close interaction between alcohol addiction and mood disorders makes complete sense when one remembers that both are connected to certain neurotransmitters in the brain such as serotonin, dopamine, norepinephrine, and so forth.

How Alcohol Affects Women Versus Men

When it comes to alcohol, there are key differences between men and women. Even small amounts of alcohol affect women differently. Women are definitely at greater risk of developing alcoholism than men, but why? For starters, women generally weigh less than men. When a woman drinks alcohol, her brain and other organs are exposed to greater concentrations of the alcohol because of fewer pounds of body weight and fewer body fluids to dilute the alcohol. The toxic effects of alcohol therefore have a greater impact on women than men.

 Question

What is fetal alcohol syndrome (FAS)?
Fetal alcohol syndrome is a collection of problems in infants caused by the mother drinking alcohol during her pregnancy. Typically, babies with FAS are born with low birth weight, distinctive abnormalities of facial features, central nervous system defects, and growth problems, and may experience brain damage resulting in problems with learning, memory, attention, and problem-solving. These problems may last a lifetime.

Specific problems with long-term alcohol addiction in women include general menstrual difficulties, the shrinking of breasts and sexual organs, and the redistribution of body fat into a pattern more typically found in men. Even one drink of alcohol per day has been found to increase the risk of breast cancer in women, especially if there is a family history of breast cancer. Alcohol consumption, with the resulting impaired judgment, slower motor responses, and so forth, can make women more vulnerable to sexual assault as well as unsafe and unplanned sex. One of the most serious consequences of a woman drinking alcohol is the potential development of fetal alcohol syndrome (FAS) in her unborn child. For this reason, it is recommended that no alcohol be consumed by a woman who is pregnant or who wants to become pregnant. Alcohol addiction is also capable of causing miscarriages. If a woman discovers she is pregnant but has already consumed alcohol, she should stop any further alcohol use immediately.

There are other interesting facts related to alcohol addiction and women. Younger women are more likely to drink heavily than older women. Women who have never been married, who are unmarried but living with a partner, and who are divorced or separated tend to drink more heavily. A woman can also be influenced by her husband—if he drinks heavily, she is also likely to drink more heavily than other women.

Reading the Signs and Symptoms

Many signs and symptoms of addiction are common to all substances of abuse. The following are signs and symptoms specific to alcohol addiction:

- Slurred or agitated speech
- Physical indications of malnutrition, such as weight loss, poor skin tone, hair loss, and so forth
- More frequent infections and illnesses
- Alcohol odors on breath or clothing
- Hidden stashes of alcohol, or alcohol disappearing
- Reports of being found intoxicated at work or school
- Social circle reduced to only those who also drink alcohol
- Alcohol used to relieve anxiety, stress, or sleep problems
- Lying or use of denial to disguise the true amount of alcohol consumed
- Use of alcohol in situations where it is dangerous to do so, such as driving, operating machinery, babysitting small children, or other situations where alertness is necessary

It may be necessary to consult a professional who specializes in assessment of addictions to sort out the many signs and symptoms that may be present. Because alcohol affects every system in the body as well as behaviors and ways of thinking, assessment of alcohol addiction can be complicated and feel overwhelming. It may even be helpful to have more than one opinion and get different perspectives from objective professionals who are knowledgeable in working with those addicted to alcohol.

Talking to a Loved One about His or Her Problem

The ideal situation for friends and family whose loved one has a problem with alcohol addiction is for the addicted individual to recognize his own problem and initiate treatment himself. If an alcohol-addicted person isn't ready to admit to his problem, it can be very frustrating for others who care about him. Friends and family members may feel helpless or even hopeless. However, there are things to do to be helpful. Don't underestimate the power of social and family influence.

Essential

State-dependent learning as related to alcoholism is a phenomenon in which a person who learns something while intoxicated will remember best when intoxicated. Once the person is sober, she will struggle to remember anything learned while intoxicated. Therefore, productive conversations are best carried out when a person is sober.

So how does one talk effectively with an alcohol-addicted person? First of all, choose the right time. The right time is when the person confronting the situation can remain calm and when the addicted person is sober. Angry and aggressive confrontations only tend to teach the alcoholic to stay away and avoid "discussions." Second, work to establish trust. This is often a key missing element in families or social circles where alcoholism is present. "Say what you mean, and mean what you say" is a worthwhile admonition to remember. Positive feedback that is direct, honest, and based in fact is helpful. The person addicted to alcohol needs to hear in a respectful, nonaggressive manner how his addiction is affecting those around him. Negative feedback that includes accusations and blame often results in the alcoholic retreating into denial and rationalization. One may feel a need to present consequences. For instance, one might state as a consequence that the alcoholic will have to clean up her own vomit. This can be effective, but make sure that no consequences are presented if there is no intent to carry through. Consequences without follow-through are only threats, and the person making the empty threats will lose credibility in future interactions.

The Road to Recovery

One has only to consider the complexities and all-encompassing effects of alcohol to know that the road to recovery is long and hard. But the goal is achievable, and the effort can be very rewarding. Recovery begins with recognizing and admitting that one definitely has a problem with alcohol.

 Question

Are there any approved medications for treating alcohol addiction?
Currently the Federal Drug Administration (FDA) has only approved three drugs for use in treating the disease of alcoholism. They are naltrexone (ReVia), acamprosate (Campral), and the anticonvulsant drug, topiramate.

For successful recovery to occur, the person addicted to alcohol must honestly acknowledge the damage done to herself and those around her as a result of the use of alcohol. Once this acknowledgement has occurred, she will recognize that the benefits of recovery outweigh the risk of continuing the addiction. Once the decision to enter recovery has been made, a person must be assessed for withdrawal symptoms. If there is any risk for delirium or seizures, medical intervention will be necessary for safety. Typically, a sedative such as diazepam (Valium), chlordiazepoxide (Librium), or lorazepam (Ativan) will be used and gradually tapered down. Propranolol (Inderal) and other beta-adrenergic blockers may be used in treating withdrawal symptoms by reducing tremors, lowering heart rate, and lowering blood pressure. Disulfiram (Antabuse) has been used historically as a deterrent to drinking. It interferes with normal metabolizing of alcohol by the liver, resulting in a toxic byproduct that leads to nausea. The cons of disulfiram are that the desire for alcohol remains after the nausea and the drug can also cause hepatitis.

If someone is dually diagnosed, other medications may be used to treat the mental illness that is present along with the alcohol addiction. Many other approaches may be used in treating alcohol addiction. Psychotherapy, behavior modification, nutritional therapy, support groups, family therapy, and other modalities may all be necessary for successful recovery. Each individual along with his treatment providers must determine which interventions will most likely lead to a life-saving recovery.

Choosing to Take the Twelve Steps

Alcoholics Anonymous (A.A.) is a self-help organization that operates worldwide. In the United States alone it is estimated that there are 1 million members. The Twelve Steps are a guide for individuals struggling with addiction and are meant to be worked on in the order presented. A.A. has a spiritual basis but does not pressure its members into accepting any particular spiritual beliefs. The only requirement for a person to join A.A. is a desire to stop drinking. According to A.A., abstinence is the only successful approach to managing alcoholism. There are no dues or financial charges to belong to A.A. and it is not associated with any other organization. A.A. meetings are run by group members, not professionals.

Many studies have been carried out in an attempt to determine the level of effectiveness in using the Twelve Steps of A.A. in the treatment of alcoholism. Results have varied, ranging from A.A. being highly effective to A.A. making no difference whatsoever. The bottom line seems to be that A.A. is quite effective for those who attend meetings regularly and commit to the process.

 Fact

Alcoholics Anonymous (A.A.) was founded in 1935 by Bill W., a stockbroker in New York City, and Dr. Bob S., a surgeon from Akron, Ohio. Both of these men suffered from severe alcoholism and had not found relief in any other treatments available at that time. Thus they formed their own self-help group based on the concept of abstinence.

The Myth of the "Dry Drunk"

The "dry drunk" is no myth at all. It is a very real syndrome that many alcoholics have to face. A dry drunk is an individual who has given up drinking alcohol, but hasn't relinquished the thoughts and behaviors that characterize an alcoholic. A dry drunk may have deceived herself that she is recovered from alcoholism, but in truth, she has only stopped drinking. Recovery from the old patterns of thinking and behaving is missing.

Essential

Family members often don't recognize the dry drunk in their midst. They may be so used to the attitudes and behaviors of the alcoholic, and so happy that the alcoholic has stopped drinking, that the signs of the dry drunk go unnoticed.

When a person with an alcohol addiction decides to enter recovery, he typically goes through a grieving process. (Grief typically includes five stages: denial, anger, bargaining, depression, and acceptance.) It is not that the individual is losing something he loves, but he is losing something with which he is very familiar. This is a painful and frightening experience. It is suggested that the dry drunk has moved through the denial stage of grief and is stuck in the anger stage.

How does one recognize a dry drunk? There is often a feeling of nostalgia for the drinking life, fantasizing or daydreaming about how things used to be. A dry drunk may act self-important and grandiose, blaming others for her problems. She may continue to engage in impulsive behaviors and impatience. There may be mood swings and feelings of dissatisfaction. The dry drunk may withdraw from others and from treatment programs, instead becoming self-absorbed and believing she can manage on her own. There is an attitude of either "poor me" or "I have all the answers." Treatment for the dry drunk involves facing the problem, completing the grief process, and continuing on with honest, genuine recovery.

CHAPTER 6

Substance Addiction

THERE ARE SO many substances available that are capable of causing addiction that it can be overwhelming and confusing to learn about each and every one. More are being developed all the time, and the new designer drugs are often variations on substances that have been available for years. However, the effort invested in becoming knowledgeable about substances of abuse is worthwhile for you and your loved ones. These drugs are dangerous and can produce lifelong harmful effects. Knowledge is one of your most powerful weapons.

Introduction to Drugs

The easiest way to begin learning about drugs of abuse and addiction is to separate them into categories. The drugs are placed into categories according to their chemical makeup and the effects they have on the body. You may recognize many of these drugs as ones that are commonly prescribed by physicians. This is not meant to be alarming. Many drugs with the potential for addiction are quite safe in doses prescribed by a physician and taken for specific medical conditions. Take the opiate category, for instance. This category contains almost all prescription pain medications. No one would think of going through a major surgical procedure with the subsequent pain without having these medications available to provide relief.

If a person understands the general characteristics of drugs in particular categories, it will be much easier to talk with professionals or other interested individuals about one's concerns.

Street names are part of a language used in the culture of substance addiction. For the uninitiated, this language is a way of communicating hidden messages related to drug use. The use of slang is especially attractive to young people, and parents need to be knowledgeable in order to monitor their children. See Appendix B for a sample list of common street names and slang related to substance addiction.

 Question

What are designer drugs?
Designer drugs are synthetic or man-made drugs. Amateur chemists change the chemical structure of existing drugs to produce different effects for the user. There are three drugs that are most commonly used as the basis for designer drugs: methamphetamine, fentanyl, and PCP. Designer drugs are very potent and extremely dangerous.

Depressants

The category of depressants should not be confused with anti-depressant medications. They are two completely different classes of drugs. Depressants act to slow down the central nervous system. In general, depressants reduce feelings of anxiety, lower inhibitions, cause drowsiness, decrease body temperature, slow down a person's pulse and breathing, and lower blood pressure. Depressants also cause confusion, problems with memory and judgment, and fatigue. They interfere with a person's ability to concentrate and exercise sound judgment. Depressants can also have serious effects on the respiratory system. It is possible for a person to experience respiratory arrest and death if that person is sensitive to the drug or if the drug is administered in high doses. Withdrawal from depressants can be very problematic. An individual may experience high levels of anxiety, insomnia, and mood swings. A small percentage of individuals may experience temporary psychosis with hallucinations and delusions. Some brand names of depressants include Amytal, Nembutal, Seconal, Phenobarbital, Ativan, Halcion, Librium, Valium, Xanax, Rohypnol, GHB (gamma-hydroxybutyrate), and Quaalude.

Cannabinoids

Marijuana and hashish are the two primary substances in this category. In general, a person using drugs from the cannabinoid category might experience euphoria as well as confusion. These drugs enhance the senses and stimulate a person's appetite.

 Alert

Individuals who smoke marijuana are at risk for developing "amotivational syndrome." Characteristics of this syndrome include lethargy and self-defeating behavior. Individuals tend to lose interest in normal activities and have been known to abandon long-term goals they were previously eager to achieve. A drop in cerebral blood flow after marijuana use seems to be the cause of amotivational syndrome.

Although someone using cannabinoids will likely feel relaxed and peaceful, the negative effects include problems with balance, coordination, memory, and learning. Lung and respiratory problems are common, including coughs and infections. Anxiety, increased heart rate, and panic attacks have also been known to occur. Many have argued that cannabinoids are not that harmful in terms of drug use. However, it is now known that cannabinoids can also lead to the development of tolerance and addiction.

Hallucinogens

Hallucinogens are also known as dissociative drugs. This is due to their ability to alter mental perceptions and thought processes. All five of the human senses can be affected by hallucinogens. A person can see things that don't exist, hear things that others don't and so forth. This has led some to believe that hallucinogens can accentuate creativity. While hallucinogens can induce pleasurable sensations, there are also many negative effects produced by hallucinogens. For example, hallucinogens can increase a person's body temperature, heart rate, and blood pressure as well as cause nausea and vomiting. Memory loss, impaired motor function, loss of appetite, insomnia, and feelings of weakness may also occur. It is important to know that this category of drugs can lead to mental health problems, including flashbacks, feelings of paranoia, hallucinations, and delusions. Some of these symptoms may last a lifetime. At times, a person may experience severe reactions to this class of drug with complete disorientation and terrifying mental images. Common hallucinogens include LSD (lysergic acid diethylamide), mescaline, PCP (phencyclidine), psilocybin (mushrooms), ketamine, and MDMA (3,4-methylenedioxymethamphetamine), otherwise known as Ecstasy.

Opiates and Morphine Derivatives

Drugs in this category may sound more familiar. Brand names of substances you may have heard before include methadone, Empirin with Codeine, Fiorinal with Codeine, Tylenol with Codeine, Duragesic, Duramorph, OxyContin, and Vicodin. Heroin and opium are also included in this category. Characteristics of these drugs are pain relief, feelings of euphoria, and sedation. They often cause drowsiness, nausea, constipation, depression, and confusion. A dangerous quality of drugs in this category is the ability to cause respiratory depression, which can lead to unconsciousness, coma, and death. An individual can definitely develop tolerance and addictions to these drugs.

Stimulants

Stimulants do exactly what the name implies—they stimulate one's body in multiple ways. Heart rate, blood pressure, body temperature, and metabolism are all increased. In fact, the heart may begin beating irregularly and heart failure may even occur. An individual affected by a stimulant will feel exhilarated and have lots of energy and perceived mental alertness. Nervousness, insomnia, reduced appetite with weight loss, paranoia, irritability, and rapid speech are all commonly experienced with drugs in this category. Amphetamines, cocaine, MDMA (3,4-methylenedioxymethamphetamine) or Ecstasy, methamphetamine, methylphenidate (Ritalin), caffeine, and nicotine are all drugs having stimulant effects.

Steroids

A different category of substances is that of anabolic steroids. The classic criteria for addiction applies to steroids. A person may continue to use them in spite of negative physical and social consequences. Withdrawal symptoms such as mood swings, fatigue, restlessness, loss of appetite, depression, problems sleeping, reduced sex drive, and the craving for more of the drug occur when use of the drug is stopped. Steroids do not induce intoxication and are not taken for the thrill of the "high." They are primarily used to enhance athletic performance. However, the side effects of steroid abuse are quite serious. High blood pressure, blood clot formation, changes in cholesterol levels, liver disease, kidney and prostate cancer, hostility and aggression, and acne only begin the list of the harmful effects of steroids. In adolescents, steroids prematurely stop physical growth of the body. Men may experience reduced sperm production, shrunken testicles, and breast enlargement. Women may develop facial hair, a deep voice, menstrual irregularities, and male-pattern baldness. The cultural and social pressures for enhanced athletic performance are very costly indeed.

 Fact

Nicotine and caffeine are stimulants, but have different chemical mechanisms than other drugs in this category. An individual who uses nicotine or caffeine is not at risk for dangerous results of overdose or the psychotic symptoms that may be seen with other stimulants.

Common Substances of Abuse

While categorizing substances of abuse is helpful for understanding and discussion, it is also true that individual substances within each category will have their own unique peculiarities. Although it is beyond the scope of this book to delve into the details of each potentially addictive substance, a closer look at two commonly known drugs would be interesting.

 Question

> **What are "club drugs?"**
> There are a number of drugs that make up the category of "club drugs." These drugs are popular with young people and are typically used in nightclubs, at parties, and at raves, which are all-night dance parties. Many drugs in this category have psychoactive, stimulant effects. Examples include MDMA (Ecstasy), ketamine, and two drugs often called "date-rape" drugs, flunitrazepam (Rohypnol) and GHB (gamma hydroxybutyrate).

Methamphetamines

Methamphetamines are very potent stimulants. These are man-made drugs rather than naturally occurring substances. Methamphetamines can be taken orally, nasally, by smoking, or by injection. They come in either a powder form or a rock form. The rock form of methamphetamines is often referred to as "crystal meth." The powerful stimulant effects of methamphetamine are due to its ability to increase the amount of dopamine available to the brain. This happens in two ways. First, methamphetamine causes the brain to release more dopamine into the space between neurons in the brain, the synaptic gap. Ordinarily, once dopamine has been used by the brain, it is reabsorbed from the synaptic gap back into the neurons, or "recycled." Second, methamphetamines increase dopamine in the brain by preventing this reabsorption, leaving excessive amounts of dopamine in the synaptic gap. In fact, methamphetamines cause a 1,500 percent increase in the brain's dopamine levels.

Initially, a person will experience a rush of energy and euphoria accompanied by compulsive behaviors, heightened senses, and a decrease in appetite. Injected or snorted methamphetamines take effect more readily than those taken orally, two to ten minutes versus twenty to forty minutes. A person may feel the effects of methamphetamines for up to twelve hours. Chronic use of methamphetamines can lead to the psychotic symptoms of auditory and visual hallucinations and/or delusions. These symptoms can last for months or even years after initial use of the drug. Paranoia and extreme rages leading to violence are especially dangerous side effects of methamphetamines. Hyperthermia (extremely high body temperature), convulsions, and even death are possible with methamphetamine use. Equally as dangerous as the side effects is the possibility of injury from the home manufacture of methamphetamines. The chemicals used in the manufacture of methamphetamines are flammable, explosive, and toxic to humans.

 Fact

Methamphetamines are also legitimately used to treat narcolepsy and attention deficit hyperactivity disorder. When used for medical purposes, methamphetamines are produced in well-supervised laboratories and dispensed by physicians. Unfortunately, however, sometimes legitimately made methamphetamines are sold illegally on the streets to individuals not under a physician's care.

MDMA (3,4-methylenedioxymethamphetamine)

The commonly known name for MDMA is Ecstasy. This is a manmade or synthetic drug that contains both the stimulant qualities of methamphetamines and the hallucinogenic qualities of mescaline. This is a dangerous drug with potentially very long-term effects.

MDMA has been shown to damage neurons leading to a depletion of the neurotransmitter serotonin. Evidence of damage to serotonin nerve terminals has been found even up to seven years after use of the drug.

MDMA has also been found to cause deterioration at the synaptic gap of neurons involved in the dopaminergic system. As expected with interference of neurotransmitters involved in the regulation of moods, MDMA causes mood, appetite, and sleep disturbances. Psychological effects of MDMA include confusion, depression, and severe anxiety. Even more seriously, MDMA can cause hyperthermia resulting in liver, kidney, and cardiovascular system failure. Death is possible with the use of this drug. MDMA is a popular "party drug" because of its production of euphoria lasting four to six hours and relatively low financial cost.

 Alert

Flunitrazepam (Rohypnol) and gamma hydroxybutyrate (GHB) are two more substances that are popular with young people at parties. Both of these substances are tasteless and odorless. They have the ability to cause sedation and intoxication as well. The combination of these characteristics has led to their use in committing sexual assaults and has earned them the title of "date-rape" drugs.

How the Body Reacts

All substances of abuse and addiction have certain qualities in common. They all bind or attach to one or more brain proteins and they all alter the functioning of brain cell receptors or neurotransmitters. As previously discussed, dopamine is the primary neurotransmitter involved in the addictive process. All addictive substances seem to hook into the dopamine pleasure pathway in some manner. This results in very pleasurable feelings and behaviors that lead to cravings for more and more of the drug. Normal physiological processes that are ordinarily rewarding, such as eating and sex, are often bypassed for the more intense responses resulting from the use of addictive substances. As the brain acclimates to the changes brought about by introducing an addictive substance into its normal functioning, the substance becomes necessary to maintain the new level of homeostasis, or balance. When the substance is stopped, uncomfortable or even dangerous withdrawal symptoms follow and cravings demand that the use of the substance be resumed.

 Fact

> Addictive substances can be detected by laboratory examination of hair, urine, sweat, saliva, and blood samples. Substances can be detected from one day up to four weeks after use. Detection times depend on the body sample used, the substance, the duration of use, and methods used, among other factors.

All addictive substances have harmful effects on the brain. However, the routes of action may be different for varying substances. For example, opiates, cannabinoids, nicotine, benzodiazepines, and hallucinogens primarily affect specific receptors. Remember, receptors are the part of the neuron that receives neurotransmitters as they are transported about the brain. Cocaine, amphetamines, Ritalin, nicotine, and marijuana in particular inhibit the reuptake or reabsorption of dopamine and thus leave an excessive quantity of dopamine in the synaptic gap. Substances in the stimulant category affect norepinephrine and serotonin uptake and alter the activity of NMDA receptors. Uptake refers to the absorption through receptors on the receiving neuron. Opiates connect directly to opiate receptors and mimic the actions of the body's own natural opiate substances—enkephalins and endorphins. Hallucinogens work through changing the serotonin and glutamine delivery systems while depressants primarily affect GABA. As one can readily see, the interactions of addictive substances with the chemicals and physiology of the brain are intricate and complex.

Knowing the Signs and Symptoms

Many signs and symptoms of substance addiction are the same as those already mentioned for alcohol addiction—the mood swings, problems in relationships, secretive behaviors or lying, changes in school or work habits, sleeping and eating problems, and so forth. Certain substances of abuse will have some of their own unique signs to watch for.

Signs and symptoms of marijuana and hashish include problems with memory, red eyes and dilated pupils, poor coordination, difficulty concentrating, increased appetite, anxiety, paranoia, and lack of motivation. Depressants may lead to the following signs and symptoms: drowsiness, depression, dizziness, poor memory, slurred speech, confusion, poor coordination, and slowed breathing. With the stimulants, one might look for a decrease in appetite, rapid speech, irritability, weight loss, paranoia, insomnia, aggressive or impulsive behavior, nasal congestion if the substance is taken nasally, exhilarated mood followed by depression as the substance wears off. An individual who uses hallucinogens might appear to have a distorted sense of reality—changes in sensory perceptions, confusion, and even an altered self-image—along with a heightened awareness of his environment. He may also experience nausea and vomiting, memory problems, impaired motor function such as tremors, panic symptoms, paranoia, hallucinations, and flashbacks. Opiates and narcotics might produce slowed breathing, constipation, depression, confusion, nausea, drowsiness, and a decreased reaction to pain. One might also notice needle marks if the substance has been injected. Of course, this also raises the possibility of infection and the symptoms that go along with that, such as redness, swelling, and fever.

The signs and symptoms of designer drugs such as Ecstasy are more difficult to predict, as the makeup of these substances can change somewhat with each batch. However, some general signs to watch for are chills and sweating, clenched teeth, drooling, loss of appetite, nausea and vomiting, memory problems, seizures, uncontrolled shaking, confusion, irrational thinking, irritability, severe anxiety, and possibly violent behavior. Inhalants (discussed in Chapter 1) are gaseous substances typically obtained through common household products. Signs and symptoms that someone may be using inhalants include inebriation, confusion, nausea, and vomiting. Individuals using inhalants may progress into stupor, unconsciousness, and even death.

 Question

What are flashbacks?
Flashbacks are perceptual experiences that may result from the use of hallucinogenic substances such as LSD. Drug flashbacks are often described as bright flashes of lights and colors. They happen when the person is no longer under the influence of the drug. In fact, flashbacks from LSD have been known to occur even as long as five years after the drug was used.

The Criminal Element

Substance addiction can become very expensive, and the consequences of substance addiction can make it very difficult for an addict to maintain successful employment. Therefore, it is not uncommon that such a person may turn to crime to support her addiction. Additionally, the illicit production and transport of illegal addictive substances is very lucrative and attracts many people involved in criminal activities who want to cash in on big profits.

It has been reported that incarcerated individuals with substance addictions are more likely than other criminals to become repeat offenders. This makes sense when one considers the strong physiological pull substances have on a person. Cravings and the desire to avoid withdrawal symptoms can relentlessly drive a person to obtain his substance of choice, sometimes even at the high cost of crime. Another problem for incarcerated individuals is the paucity of substance abuse treatment. Only a very small percentage of individuals needing substance abuse treatment in jail actually receive it. Drug-related crimes are typically theft, manufacturing and selling illegal substances, and public disturbances related to drug trafficking and use. Unfortunately, there also are many drug-related crimes that involve violence with resulting injury or death. Substance addiction education and treatment could be two of the most effective deterrents to crime in our society.

 Fact

According to a U.S. Department of Justice report released in 2004, 17 percent of state prisoners and 18 percent of federal prisoners admitted they committed their current offense to obtain money for drugs. Thirty-two percent of state prisoners and 26 percent of federal prisoners admitted they were under the influence of drugs when they committed their current crimes.

Talking to a Loved One about His or Her Problem

Remember that the addicted person has a disease. Substance addiction can alter one's thinking and perceptions of reality. Therefore, it is necessary to do one's homework before talking to a friend or loved one about her substance abuse problem.

If you suspect that the person you want to talk with is using a particular substance, learn all you can from reading this book and others about how that substance affects one's physical and mental state. Know the signs and symptoms. Research various treatment facilities that treat that particular substance addiction so that you can make knowledgeable recommendations if appropriate. Angry, aggressive confrontations are unlikely to be effective. Concern expressed firmly but lovingly will likely gain the most beneficial results. Let your friend or loved one know what you are willing to do to help (e.g., babysitting or providing transportation to treatment).

You will recall that it is common for an addicted individual to be in denial. Sometimes he is in denial about being addicted, but he may also be in denial about his addiction affecting others in negative ways. It is important that the addicted person be made aware of how his actions affect those around him. A well-thought-out letter that describes factual incidents in a nonaccusatory manner may be helpful and gives the addicted person time to ponder the effects of his addiction without feeling pressured. Many addicted persons have low self-esteem and could be resistant to getting treatment for themselves. However, they may be willing to enter treatment to protect the ones they love.

 Alert

Safety is a primary concern in talking with a friend or loved one about substance addiction. Some substances such as methamphetamines can cause irrational, aggressive, or violent behaviors. Be prepared for this possibility, and don't hesitate to call 911 if there is a need.

Formal family interventions are controversial. They may produce further resistance from the addicted person if he feels attacked or humiliated in front of others. Current thinking is that motivational interviewing is more effective in working with an addicted person. Motivational interviewing is a lighter form of confrontation and is conducted by a licensed therapist. It is done in a one-on-one setting with the therapist encouraging an addicted person to explore any ambivalence he may have about his addiction. The therapist supports him with empathy, understanding, and objective feedback. Rather than intervene yourself, you might do research to locate a qualified therapist trained in this technique.

Overcoming Substance Addiction

The most important first step in overcoming addiction is to ensure safe withdrawal or detoxification from the addictive substance. This may be possible on an outpatient basis, but if withdrawal symptoms are severe, inpatient treatment may be necessary. In either case, medical supervision of the withdrawal period is recommended. Different categories of substances will have different withdrawal symptoms and therefore require different approaches.

L.₌ Essential

There are many alternative methods available to treat withdrawal symptoms, such as herbal remedies, acupuncture, nutritional therapy, and psychic healing. Although some of these methods may be quite helpful, research is limited as to safety and effectiveness. Always consult a physician trained in treating substance addictions to help make wise choices regarding a treatment regimen.

Withdrawal from opiates in particular can be very difficult. Symptoms of opiate withdrawal may resemble severe influenza, with runny nose, coughing, diarrhea, nausea, and vomiting. The potential dehydration resulting from these symptoms needs to be aggressively treated. Individuals undergoing a planned medical withdrawal from opiates may be administered buprenorphine or methadone as they taper off the addictive substance. Clonidine is a medication often given to help relieve severe anxiety symptoms that may accompany withdrawal.

Symptoms of withdrawal seen in individuals addicted to depressants include restlessness, anxiety, sleep problems, and sweating. It is possible to develop hallucinations, seizures, increased blood pressure, heart rate, and body temperature. Delirium may also develop and is potentially life-threatening. Tapering off the drug gradually is one way of managing withdrawal from depressants. Medical treatment is definitely needed for more serious symptoms.

Withdrawal from stimulants often induces fatigue, anxiety, depression, and intense cravings. Suicidal thoughts and attempts, paranoia, and acute psychosis are possible, requiring inpatient treatment for safety. Physicians may prescribe antidepressant and/or antipsychotic medications to treat symptoms.

Remember, withdrawal from any addictive substance must be taken seriously. One can see that symptoms can range from mildly uncomfortable to life-threatening. Factors determining severity of withdrawal symptoms include the individual physical makeup of the addict, the properties of the addictive substance itself, the amount of substance consumed, the length of time the person was addicted, and complications such as coexisting medical problems, other mental health disorders, or dealing with multiple addictive substances.

In addition to managing withdrawal, treatment of substance addiction may involve inpatient hospitalization, partial hospitalization, outpatient therapy and/or self-help support groups. These treatment modalities utilize individual and family therapy, cognitive-behavior therapy, and education designed to help an addict manage his cravings and prevent relapse.

Rehab and Recovery

Rehabilitation and recovery really are about getting cravings under control and preventing relapse. They are also about learning coping skills to better manage life stressors, emotions, and interpersonal relationships. In the early stages of recovery, it is also important to identify triggers that might precipitate a relapse. Old friends who were partners in substance use, places where substance use took place, and other reminders will need to be avoided. Developing structure in one's daily life is helpful in keeping focused on rehabilitation and recovery. In severe cases of substance addiction, residential rehabilitation programs may be beneficial in providing a safe, contained, therapeutic, and supportive environment while getting started on the road to successful recovery. Support is essential, as very few people are able to successfully recover from substance addiction alone. Twelve-step groups are one type of support system especially designed for recovering addicts. The support of family and friends is certainly important, but most addicted persons feel that the understanding and support they receive from others who have experienced similar problems is essential to maintaining recovery.

CHAPTER 7

Nicotine Addiction

NICOTINE HAS COME a long way from the glamorous depictions of smoking in the movies and advertisements of the early to mid-twentieth century. It is now recognized for what it really is, a killer of millions of Americans through cancers, lung diseases, and heart disease. Smoking is the leading preventable cause of death in this country. However, be encouraged. Even a person who has used nicotine products for many years can reverse much of the damage by abstaining from use of these addictive substances and engaging in healthy lifestyle habits.

Got a Light?

The chemical nicotine was first identified from the tobacco plant in the early 1800s. Although it is the key ingredient in tobacco, there are over 4,000 additional substances in tobacco and tobacco smoke that affect one's body. At least sixty of those additional substances are known to cause cancer. Nicotine is a highly addictive substance and is the chemical in tobacco products that keeps one asking for more. However, it may not be the only addictive substance in tobacco. Scientists have recently discovered that acetaldehyde, a chemical found in tobacco smoke, enhances the addictive properties of nicotine.

How does a person know if she is addicted to nicotine? The signs and symptoms are certainly similar to other addictive substances. She has likely attempted to quit smoking unsuccessfully many times. As many as 85 percent of individuals who smoke claim they want to quit. However, the success rate of quitting smoking without help is only 5 to 6 percent. Strong and specific withdrawal symptoms occur when a person stops using nicotine. The health problems caused by tobacco products are well publicized, yet an addicted individual continues to use the substance in spite of that knowledge. She would not likely spend excessive amounts of time and money to obtain nicotine products, as they are readily available. However, she may give up social and/or recreational activities in favor of smoking.

Fact

Adolescence is the most common time in life to begin smoking. It has been suggested that 90 percent of smokers began their addiction prior to age twenty-one. This raises concern that an individual who begins smoking in adolescence is more likely to become a heavily addicted smoker in adulthood.

Several aspects are different for nicotine than for other addictive substances. Remember that tolerance is defined as the need for an increasing amount of a substance in order to achieve the desired effect. With nicotine, tolerance is defined as an absence of nausea, dizziness, and other symptoms of beginning usage despite an increasing intake of the substance. Also, while intoxication is often a goal in the use of other addictive products, a person does not become intoxicated with nicotine.

Alert

Nicotine usage reached a peak in the mid-1990s. Since that time, there has been a decline in nicotine addiction. However, in recent years the rate of decline in nicotine usage is slowing, suggesting that renewed efforts to educate children and adolescents in particular are essential if there is to be a continuing drop in the use of this highly addictive and dangerous substance.

Nicotine is most commonly associated with cigarettes. Additionally, smokeless tobacco products are also commonplace. The two most common types of smokeless tobacco are chewing tobacco and snuff. Chewing tobacco comes in the form of loose leaves, plugs, or twists of tobacco. Chewing tobacco may be referred to in the slang terms of "plugs," "wads," or "chew." It is literally chewed or placed between the gums and cheeks. An individual sucks out the nicotine and then spits out the tobacco juices. The nicotine is absorbed through the tissues of the mouth. Snuff is finely ground tobacco and also comes in various forms: dry, moist, or in sachets. It can be sniffed or inhaled through the nose, or moist snuff is pinched off and placed between the lower lip or cheek and gum. Smokeless tobacco is less lethal than cigarettes, but also contains cancer-causing chemicals and can end in addiction. Adolescents who begin their nicotine addiction with smokeless tobacco are more likely to progress on to cigarettes. Less popular but still available and used are tobacco lozenges marketed as Ariva and Stonewall.

 Question

What is snus?
Snus (pronounced "snoose") is moist snuff that is commonly used in Sweden and Norway. The marketing pitch for snus is that it reportedly has fewer cancer-causing agents than other smokeless tobacco products. But don't be fooled. It is not harmless and still has serious health risks. Snus has also been introduced into the United States.

In 2004, it was said that 22 percent of American high school students and 12 percent of middle school students smoked tobacco. Although the percentages of young people who use tobacco had declined since the 1990s, this decline has now leveled off. The negative health and economic impact that this highly addictive substance has had on the United States is phenomenal.

The Physiological Effects of Nicotine

What makes nicotine so dangerous and so addictive? Again, the answer begins in the brain. When a person takes a puff on a cigarette, the nicotine is pulled into the lungs and absorbed directly into the bloodstream. Within eight to ten seconds, nicotine has penetrated the brain and begins to cause its characteristic "rush."

Nicotine and the Brain

A logical question is, how could the brain be affected so quickly? Part of the answer has to do with the shape of the nicotine molecule. Its shape is similar to a natural neurotransmitter in the brain called acetylcholine. Because the shape of nicotine is so close to that of acetylcholine, it can fit into the receptor sites on brain cells that actually belong to acetylcholine. One might think of nicotine as an interloper in the brain's messenger system. Once nicotine has connected with the acetylcholine receptors, a person's heart rate, blood pressure, and respirations increase as does the release of glucose into the bloodstream. The person smoking may experience these changes and interpret them as increased mental alertness.

 Fact

Depression among smokers is three times more common than with nonsmokers. Thus it is thought that many individuals use nicotine as a way to self-medicate their mood disorder. Individuals who are treated with medication and therapy for their depression are more likely to successfully quit smoking and remain smoke-free.

Another way that nicotine affects the brain is through the now familiar dopamine pleasure pathway. Nicotine stimulates the release of large amounts of dopamine, the neurotransmitter that causes intense feelings of pleasure. You may recall from reading about methamphetamines in Chapter 6 that once dopamine has completed its prescribed function of transmitting messages from neuron to neuron, in a normally functioning brain it gets recycled. For some unknown reason, components of cigarette smoke block the reabsorption of dopamine. It remains in the space between the neurons called the synaptic gap, contributing to the intense feelings of pleasure that a person addicted to nicotine experiences. Beta-endorphins are another type of neurotransmitter that have the ability to enhance moods. Nicotine stimulates the release of beta-endorphins as well as dopamine. In addition to these significant effects of nicotine on one's brain, it also has been found to interrupt the flow of oxygen to the brain, especially the right hemisphere. Nicotine also elevates the body's levels of cortisol, which is a hormone involved in relieving stress by arousing the sympathetic nervous system.

 Alert

Research has shown that adolescents who smoke are fifteen times more likely than nonsmoking peers to experience anxiety, depression, and panic attacks. One possible explanation is that nicotine may damage blood vessels to the brain while also decreasing oxygenation to the lungs. This is yet one more reason why it is so important to educate young people about nicotine use.

One can readily see that nicotine affects the brain on many levels. However, these effects come and go quickly. Recall that the drug reaches the brain within eight to ten seconds. Within forty minutes, half of the effects caused by nicotine are over. This process is somewhat slower for a person who uses smokeless tobacco or who smokes cigars or pipes. The result is that, before long, someone addicted to nicotine is needing another dose of the drug either to achieve the desired effects or to prevent withdrawal symptoms. Over a period of time, the brain begins to make changes in order to adjust to the effects of the drug, particularly the increased production of dopamine. For example, the brain cuts down on its normal production of dopamine and reduces the number of certain brain cell receptors. Again, adjustments must be made to maintain homeostasis, or balance, in the brain's functioning. The addicted person must now consume more of the drug to stimulate the release of more dopamine just to feel "normal." Failure to use nicotine again leads to very unpleasant withdrawal effects. Withdrawal symptoms will typically appear within twenty-four hours of stopping nicotine use. Specific nicotine withdrawal symptoms include a depressed mood, problems with sleeping, irritability or anger, anxiety, problems with concentration, restlessness, a decreased heart rate, and an increase in appetite with weight gain.

Systemic Effects of Nicotine

While much attention has been given to the effects of nicotine on the brain, nicotine has harmful effects on every vital organ in the body. In the lungs, nicotine is a primary contributor to lung cancer, emphysema, pneumonia, and chronic bronchitis. Nicotine has been connected to leukemia and cataracts. It has been strongly associated with cancers of the esophagus, larynx, throat, mouth, bladder, pancreas, liver, kidneys, cervix, stomach, colon, and rectum. The heart and circulatory systems demonstrate the harmful effects of nicotine through strokes, heart attacks, vascular diseases, and aneurysms. In terms of the reproductive system, nicotine increases the risks for infertility and miscarriages in women and impotence and infertility in men. Infants are at risk for low birth weight, premature delivery, and lung problems when their mothers use nicotine during their pregnancies. Smoking tends to deaden one's sense of taste and smell, which can contribute to poor appetite and a loss of enjoyment while eating. The immune system is affected and individuals addicted to nicotine seem to be more prone to infectious illnesses such as colds and the flu compared to nonaddicted people. Smoking tends to dry and irritate one's skin cells, promoting wrinkles and giving one the appearance of premature aging.

Cigarette smoking can also cause a yellowing of one's teeth, fingers, and fingernails. Smokeless tobacco products can cause gum disease, bad breath, and stained teeth. They can also destroy the bone sockets surrounding one's teeth and thus cause tooth loss. The number of harmful effects from nicotine can definitely be overwhelming and frightening. There is hope, and treatment options will be discussed soon. But first, consider the psychological aspects of nicotine addiction.

 Question

What is nicotine poisoning?
Nicotine poisoning occurs when someone is exposed to high levels of nicotine. It only takes one drop of pure nicotine to cause death. Symptoms of nicotine poisoning include vomiting, tremors, convulsions, and even death. One way this may occur is through exposure to high doses of insecticides that contain nicotine. It does not occur from smoking too much.

The Psychological Component

Depression and anxiety are common accompaniments of nicotine addiction. Some believe that nicotine is used to self-medicate preexisting mental disorders, but it is also clear that depression and anxiety also result from the addiction. This is especially true during times of withdrawal. It has been clearly demonstrated that nicotine addiction is two to four times more prevalent in individuals with mental disorders such as post-traumatic stress disorder (PTSD), bipolar disorder, major depression, and so on, than in the general population. In fact, people with schizophrenia reportedly have a nicotine addiction rate of 90 percent. This is not to imply that nicotine causes mental illness, but rather that a person may use nicotine to cope with the uncomfortable symptoms of mental illness.

A major psychological component of nicotine addiction is the associations between the substance and the environment. Places, people, and circumstances may become closely tied with the pleasurable feelings of nicotine in one's mind. A person might mentally go through every step of the process of "lighting up"—placing the cigarette between the fingers, lighting the match, inhaling the first puff, and so forth. The addiction is intensified by the habits that are developed in conjunction with use. A person may associate smoking with the day's first cup of coffee, with reading the newspaper, with visiting a certain friend, with driving to work, etc. The memories of these events combined with the "rush" sensation of nicotine are very powerfully reinforcing.

Essential

Even newborns whose mothers smoked during pregnancy may experience signs of stress and withdrawal symptoms. Children born to nicotine-addicted mothers are also more likely to develop learning and behavioral problems. If these children begin to smoke themselves later on, they are twice as likely as children from nonaddicted mothers to develop a nicotine addiction.

The Dangers of Secondhand Smoke

Secondhand smoke is also referred to as environmental smoke. A person is exposed to secondhand smoke when she breathes in the smoke given off at the burning end of a cigarette and the smoke exhaled by a smoker. Someone who breathes secondhand smoke is said to be passively or involuntarily smoking. More than 4,000 chemicals have been identified in secondhand smoke. At least fifty of these chemicals are known to cause cancer, including arsenic, benzene, cadmium, chromium, nickel, and vinyl chloride.

Secondhand smoke can cause many of the same health problems as the direct use of nicotine. It is particularly dangerous for children, whose lungs may not be fully developed. Children exposed to secondhand smoke are at increased risk for sudden infant death syndrome (SIDS), ear infections, colds, pneumonia, bronchitis, asthma, coughs, wheezing, breathlessness, and retarded growth of the lungs. Thus far, research has found no safe levels of secondhand smoke—even the lowest doses of exposure can be harmful.

Alert

According to the National Cancer Institute, approximately 3,000 nonsmoker deaths per year due to lung cancer are attributed to secondhand smoke exposure. It has been estimated that living with a smoker increases a nonsmoker's risk of developing lung cancer by 20 to 30 percent.

Steps are being taken to protect the air for nonsmokers on local, state, and federal levels. In many locations around the country, public workplaces, restaurants, bars, and meeting places are now declared nonsmoking areas. Nationally, smoking is prohibited on domestic airline flights, most international airline flights, interstate buses, and most trains. Unfortunately, the response from tobacco companies has been to focus their advertising campaigns more on smokeless tobacco products. They present smokeless tobacco products as attractive alternatives for nicotine-addicted individuals to use in places where smoking is no longer allowed.

The Most Difficult Addiction to Break?

Many individuals with multiple addictions would argue that nicotine is the most difficult addiction to stop. Whether this is true or not is unknown. What is known is that nicotine is indeed highly addictive, equal in addictive qualities to heroin or cocaine. Even though nicotine delivers its pleasurable effects quickly, the byproducts of nicotine, such as cotinine, stay in a person's system for three to four days. When someone stops smoking, the withdrawal symptoms are quite unpleasant and cravings can last for weeks, months, or longer.

As wholeheartedly as someone might want to stop her nicotine addiction, the discomfort from withdrawal and the intense cravings caused by both physiological and psychological processes often send her back to the addiction. She might find that it takes multiple attempts to finally be nicotine-free. This is not meant to be discouraging, but rather the opposite. If a person is not successful on his first attempt to stop his nicotine addiction, he should not give up, but persevere to successful recovery.

Essential

As difficult as it is to stop a nicotine addiction, there are good reasons to do so. Within twenty-four hours of stopping use, a person's blood pressure and risk for heart attack decrease. The longer a person is nicotine-free, the greater the health benefits such as decreased risk of stroke, cancers, and lung diseases. It has been said that if a man stops smoking before he reaches thirty-five years of age, he will add approximately five years to his life expectancy.

Talking to a Loved One about His or Her Problem

It is very important in talking to a friend or loved one about his nicotine addiction that you affirm to him that he is a person you care about even though you don't like the addiction. As mentioned before, nicotine addiction has some side effects that are unpleasant to those around the addict—spitting, bad breath, yellowed fingers and fingernails, discolored teeth, aging skin, smoke odor that clings to his clothes—as well as the mess made by ashes and cigarette butts. It would be easy to focus on these outward signs, but this leads to shame and self-consciousness rather than recovery. In light of the serious health risks to someone you care about, these issues are minimal. That doesn't mean that you can't discuss how the addict's behaviors affects others. You should be honest and firm, but caring and genuinely concerned for the addicted person.

Encourage your friend or loved one to seek help from a physician knowledgeable in treating nicotine addiction. You may provide him with information to read regarding current treatments that are available. When eating out or socializing, take him to nonsmoking restaurants and clubs. The smell of others smoking may trigger cravings. This also helps to normalize a nonsmoking lifestyle. Allow your friend or loved one to talk about her problem without condemnation. There are always strong feelings connected with stopping addictions that need a healthy outlet.

 Fact

Research reported in 2006 for the Society for the Study of Addiction connected nicotine dependence with compulsive alcohol cravings. It is well known that an addicted person often has multiple addictions. This research makes it clear that shared physiological mechanisms of addiction and cravings make it more difficult for someone to stop alcohol addiction if they are also addicted to nicotine.

Treatment Options

There are now numerous treatment options available to help someone stop his nicotine addiction. Primarily, treatment falls into the categories of behavioral therapy, support groups, nicotine replacement, and other pharmacological treatments.

Behavioral Therapy

At one time, formal smoking-cessation programs offered privately or in public health settings were quite popular. Though still available, they are often time-limited due both to the structure of the program and financial considerations. This may be a good strategy to begin treatment, but additional behavioral treatment may be needed to increase the chances of successful recovery. Additional treatment can be obtained from a qualified therapist trained in treating addictions or even through the Internet or over the telephone.

The U.S. Department of Health and Human Services established a national toll-free telephone number in 2004 (800-QUIT-NOW or 800-784-8669) to help nicotine-addicted individuals gather information and quit smoking. A website has also been created (*www.smokefree .gov*) to provide online advice about quitting smoking. Almost all behavioral smoking-cessation treatments, whether formalized or not, focus on teaching the addicted person how to recognize triggers, the development of coping strategies and problem-solving skills, stress management, and how to engage social support.

 Question

Are alternative medicine approaches helpful?
Alternative medicine approaches to smoking-cessation include acupuncture, hypnosis, and guided-imagery. Although some people have claimed that they found these methods helpful, the reviews are definitely mixed. Research does not support any of these methods as clearly beneficial above other treatments for nicotine addiction.

Support Groups

Nicotine Anonymous is the primary support group targeting nicotine addiction. This group is based on the Twelve Steps of A.A., as are other groups of this nature. Support groups can also be accessed online. Additionally, telephone counseling and support systems have been set up to help a person recover from nicotine addiction. These are often offered by one's insurance company. Another program of this type offered by the American Cancer Society is Quitline Tobacco Cessation Program. Information can be obtained by calling the American Cancer Society at 800-ACS-2345. The support of family and friends may be the most helpful support group of all.

Nicotine Replacement Treatments

In general, nicotine replacement treatments provide minimal levels of nicotine to help an addicted person gradually cut down and finally quit. The nicotine found in this type of treatment has fewer severe physiological effects than tobacco and has little abuse potential. Nicotine replacement treatments do not contain the carcinogens and gases associated with tobacco products including smokeless tobacco. They come in both prescription and nonprescription products. Prescription products include a nicotine nasal spray (brand name Nicotrol NS) and a nicotine inhaler (Nicotrol inhaler). A person needs to be under the treatment of a physician to obtain these products. Nonprescription treatments can be obtained in one's local pharmacy; they include the nicotine patch (Nicoderm CQ, Nicotrol, Habitrol, and others), nicotine gum (Nicorette and others), and a nicotine lozenge (Commit).

Essential

Even though many nicotine addiction treatment products may be obtained without a prescription, they do come in different dosages with recommended time frames for treatment. It can still be helpful to consult a physician for advice on the most effective way to use these products.

Other Pharmacological Treatments

Remember that nicotine interferes with the dopamine system in the brain, affecting one's moods. The FDA has approved an antidepressant medication, buproprion (Zyban) to help a person quit smoking. Another antidepressant that has also been used in treating nicotine addiction is nortriptyline (Aventyl, Pamelor). Varenicline tartrate (Chantix) is another type of medication that acts directly on the receptor sites in the brain affected by nicotine. This drug reduces the feelings of pleasure derived from smoking as well as decreases withdrawal symptoms. Finally, a nicotine vaccine (NicVAX) may soon be available. It is still in clinical trials. This vaccine is designed to stimulate the development of antibodies to nicotine. These antibodies would prevent nicotine from accessing the brain and reinforcing its further use. This is an exciting new possibility for those who struggle with nicotine addiction. All of these products require treatment by a physician.

CHAPTER 8

Prescription Drug Addiction

THE DISCOVERY AND development of a wide array of prescription medications has been a tremendous blessing. They have made the pain of surgery, serious injuries, and chronic illnesses bearable. Stimulant medications have helped children and adults conquer the symptoms of ADHD and enjoy success in school and work. Medications for sleep disorders and anxiety have made it possible for individuals to experience some peace in their lives and get badly needed rest. However, there can be a dark side to these medications—the possibility of addiction.

But the Doctor Prescribed It!

Prescription drugs are safe for most people provided they are used in the correct dosage and for the purpose prescribed by the physician. The key to safe use is professional supervision. There are three classes of prescription drugs that are commonly abused and may become addictive: opiates, central nervous system (CNS) depressants, and stimulants. More details will come on the specific drugs involved, but for now the question is, why would any drug with the potential for addiction be prescribed? Opiates are also known as prescription narcotics and are primarily used for their pain-relieving properties. The pain associated with surgeries, dental work, serious injuries, and certain chronic illnesses is greatly alleviated through the use of prescription narcotics. Some drugs in this category are also helpful in treating coughs and diarrhea.

CNS depressants are also known as sedatives and tranquilizers. They tend to slow down normal brain functioning and, because of this property, they have been found to effectively treat anxiety, acute stress, panic attacks, and sleep disorders. The medical use of stimulants has shifted over the years. In times past, stimulants were used to treat asthma, obesity, neurological disorders, and so forth. Once the addictive nature of stimulants became apparent, their use was significantly curtailed. Now stimulants are primarily used only for treating ADHD, narcolepsy, and depression that has not responded to more typical antidepressant treatments. It is important to remember that when these medications are used as prescribed, very few individuals develop addictions.

 Fact

Even over-the-counter (OTC) medications can be abused when not used as directed. Cough suppressants, sleep aids, antihistamines, and antinausea medications may have psychoactive effects when used in excess. When combined with alcohol, OTC medications can be especially dangerous. Follow the directions carefully on the labels and call a doctor if harmful side effects become apparent.

When the Risks Outweigh the Benefits

Prescription drugs have legitimate reasons for being used and this should not be overlooked simply because they can become addictive. Of course, caution is in order, particularly for an individual who has previously struggled with addictions. You will recall that addictions often run in families and there are likely genetic components to how the brain processes substances with potentially addictive properties. Someone with the propensity to addictions as noted through family history, or someone who has previously been addicted to non-medical substances and/or compulsive behaviors, should be very cautious when using prescription medications that could become addictive when abused.

Does this mean these medications can't ever be used? No. Surgery for a broken arm, the pain from cancer, or severe panic attacks, for example, create medical necessity for the use of prescriptive drugs with addictive potential. Nevertheless, for an individual at risk, close medical monitoring by a physician knowledgeable about addictions will be necessary.

 Alert

> Prescription drug addiction is now second only to marijuana in terms of being the most abused substance in the United States. Approximately 7 million Americans abused prescription drugs in 2006. This was greater than the number of people abusing cocaine, heroin, and Ecstasy combined.

At-Risk Populations

Other populations have also been identified as "at risk" for addiction to prescription medications. What does it mean to be "at risk" for addictions? In general, a person who is "at risk" for addiction is someone who has a special interest in or is drawn toward an addictive substance, such as someone with chronic pain or someone who suffers from a mental illness. It could be someone with a genetic predisposition or someone whose environment is heavily influenced with addictive substances and behaviors. An "at risk" person is likely someone with easy access. It may be someone who has experimented with an addictive substance, experienced the initial rush of pleasure, and is then tempted to further use.

The elderly is one population that is "at risk" for prescription drug addiction. As our senior population grows, so do chronic illnesses and broken bones. The elderly are three times more likely to be taking prescription medications than other people, are less likely to understand and follow directions, and are more likely to be taking multiple medications for longer periods of time. As a person ages, the body begins to metabolize drugs differently. Typically, there is a decrease in the percentage of water and lean tissue in the body along with an increase in fat. The kidneys and liver function less efficiently. These changes affect how long a drug stays in the body and how much is actually absorbed into the body's tissues. If this isn't taken into account by medical professionals or if a person doesn't follow instructions carefully, serious harmful consequences can result. Benzodiazepines, used to treat anxiety disorders, can be particularly hazardous in the elderly if misused, possibly leading to cognitive impairment.

Essential

Prescription drugs are now the most commonly abused drug among twelve- to thirteen-year-olds. The recreational use of pain medications such as Vicodin and Percodan as well as the stimulant Ritalin is alarmingly on the rise. Education and supervision is essential to curb this trend.

Women, especially young women in their teen years and early twenties, are at greater risk for addiction to prescription drugs than men. The nonmedical use of prescription medications among women may be attributed to the social pressure to lose weight, a desire to increase self-confidence, a way of coping with problems, and a means of reducing tension. For women, there may be less social stigma in using prescription medications than street drugs. Statistics show that men and boys are more likely to become dependent on street drugs and alcohol, initially for the purpose of thrill-seeking, than on prescription drugs.

Health care workers such as physicians, nurses, pharmacists, and others with easy access to prescription medications are in a position to prevent addiction but may also be "at risk."

Identifying a Problem

As with other addictions, there are signs to watch for that may indicate problems with prescription medications. Initially, this type of addiction may be more difficult to identify because use of the medication may have started out with legitimate purposes in mind. Following are some questions you might ask to determine if you have a problem with prescription drugs:

- Do you begin to wonder if you should cut down on your use of prescription drugs?
- Do you become annoyed if others comment on your use of prescription drugs?
- Do you feel guilty about taking prescription drugs?
- Do you use prescription drugs for purposes other than those prescribed?
- Do you feel shame, embarrassment, or uneasiness in asking your physician for an early prescription renewal?

Physicians and other health care professionals should be on the alert for unscheduled requests to refill prescriptions or requests for a rapid increase in dosage. Continuing to request prescriptions for potentially addictive medications when there is no longer any valid medical reason is another danger sign.

Alert

One reason for the increase in prescription drug addiction is the development of web-based pharmacies called e-pharmacies. They often illegally sell drugs without prescriptions or consultations with the patient, making it easy to obtain numerous prescription drugs. The Drug Enforcement Agency (DEA) and the Federal Drug Administration (FDA) have ongoing investigations into this practice.

"Doctor shopping" is when someone visits multiple practitioners or multiple medical facilities in an attempt to obtain as many prescriptions as possible without being detected as an addict. This is another sign that a person may be addicted to prescription medications.

Commonly Abused Prescription Drugs

Certainly any prescription drug can be misused or abused, but in terms of addictive qualities, three categories of prescription drugs stand out. Not only are these particular categories of prescription medications more potentially addictive than others, they are also more dangerous when mixed or used in combination with other types of medications.

 Fact

Opiates are the oldest known pain relievers. In fact, these drugs were available in many nonprescription, over-the-counter medications in the early part of the twentieth century. They were used for adults and children alike. It was only after problems with addiction became more apparent that these drugs became regulated by the government and available only with a prescription.

Opiates

Opiates were briefly presented in Chapter 6. As previously mentioned, opiates are primarily used to treat pain and can also be used to treat persistent coughs and diarrhea. Opiates achieve these pain-relieving effects by attaching to specific opiate receptors found in the brain, the spinal cord, and the gastrointestinal tract. Once attached to these receptors, opiates block the perception of pain. These receptors are intended for the body's naturally produced endorphins, which also reduce pain.

Opiates can also produce a sensation of euphoria by acting on the pleasure centers of the brain. When opiates are injected or snorted rather than taken orally, the feelings of euphoria are heightened. These feelings of pleasure and euphoria produced by the drugs are often used to mask emotional pain as well as physical pain. Besides their pain-relieving qualities, opiates also produce drowsiness, nausea, constipation, and depressed respirations in larger doses. Because the body can become dependent on opiates, there will likely be withdrawal symptoms when the drug is stopped. The withdrawal symptoms may begin within hours of stopping the drug and can be quite uncomfortable. Restlessness, muscle and bone pain, insomnia, diarrhea, vomiting, involuntary leg movements, cravings, runny nose, excessive sweating, yawning, and cold flashes with "goose bumps" are typical withdrawal symptoms. For opiates, medical supervision of withdrawal is recommended. Opiates should never be taken in combination with other medications that also depress the CNS. Alcohol, antihistamines, barbiturates, benzodiazepines, or general anesthetics are examples of such medications. This is because opiates can depress the respiratory system. Taking large doses of opiates or combining opiates with CNS depressant medications can be life-threatening.

 Alert

OxyContin is particularly dangerous when abused. It contains a much greater percentage of its active ingredient, oxycodone, in each pill compared to other pain relievers. When crushed or diluted with water, the addict can snort or inject the drug, obtaining powerful effects in a much shorter period of time than other drugs.

The most common examples of opiate drugs are oxycodone (Oxy-Contin, Percodan, Percocet), propoxyphene (Darvon), hydrocodone (Vicodin, Lortab, Lorcet), hydromorphone (Dilaudid), meperidine

(Demerol), diphenoxylate (Lomotil), morphine (Kadian, Avinza, MS Contin), codeine, fentanyl (Duragesic), and methadone.

CNS Depressants

The CNS is that part of the nervous system controlled by the brain and spinal cord. It is the main processing center for the body's entire nervous system. One can clearly understand how any medications affecting the CNS can have very serious consequences if used in an abusive manner. Medications in the CNS depressant category do exactly what the name implies; they depress or slow down the brain's ability to function. They do this by affecting the neurotransmitter gamma-aminobutyric acid (GABA). CNS depressants increase GABA activity in the brain, slowing it down and thereby producing a calming effect. For an individual suffering from anxiety or sleep disorders, this is very helpful. However, as with other potentially addictive drugs, CNS depressants can lead to the development of tolerance, and withdrawal symptoms can occur when the drug is stopped. Withdrawal symptoms begin when the brain "bounces back," so to speak, from its drug-induced inactivity. When this happens, the brain seems to race out of control and life-threatening seizures can occur.

⌐. Essential

It is never safe to mix medications unless under medical supervision. Even OTC medications can have harmful effects when taken in conjunction with other prescription drugs. And remember, alcohol, a potent substance on its own, can have lethal effects when taken with prescription medications, especially CNS depressants.

Less drastic symptoms can include confusion and dizziness, impaired judgment, memory problems, decreased intellectual performance, and lack of motor coordination. CNS depressants should not be combined with any other medication that has similar effects.

This includes OTC cold remedies and allergy medications. Certain herbal compounds, such as valerian and kava, may exacerbate the effects of certain CNS depressants to a dangerous level. The combination of alcohol and CNS depressants can be lethal.

The CNS depressant category includes barbiturates and benzodiazepines. Medications known as barbiturates are mephobarbital (Mebaral) and pentobarbital sodium (Nembutal). Benzodiazepines include diazepam (Valium), chlordiazepoxide hydrochloride (Librax), chlordiazepoxide (Librium), alprazolam (Xanax), triazolam (Halcion), estazolam (ProSom), clonazepam (Klonopin), and lorazepam (Ativan).

 Question

Why are stimulants used to treat attention deficit hyperactivity disorder (ADHD)?
ADHD is a disorder in which the norepinephrine and dopamine transport systems are defective, leading to a deficit in the available amount of these neurotransmitters. Norepinephrine and dopamine work in the prefrontal cortex and the striatum of the brain to help promote informational processing, working memory, and self-control. Stimulants inhibit the reabsorption of these neurotransmitters, making them more available for use.

Stimulants

Just as CNS depressants depress brain activity, stimulants stimulate the brain. They enhance one's sense of alertness, attention, and energy. Stimulants also increase a person's blood pressure, heart rate, blood glucose, and respirations. Sleep deprivation and a suppressed appetite may also result from stimulant use. The effects of stimulants are due to their enhancement of norepinephrine and dopamine in the brain. You will recall that dopamine is responsible for the pleasure circuit in the brain. Based on that fact, you won't be surprised to learn that stimulants can also produce feelings of euphoria and pleasure. Stimulants are primarily used to treat narcolepsy, ADHD, and treatment resistant depression. In times past, stimulants were considered effective treatments for asthma, obesity, neurological problems, and so forth. However, their medical use has diminished because of their addictive nature.

Stopping the use of stimulants also leads to withdrawal symptoms. Fatigue, depression, and disturbed sleep patterns are common. Hostility or paranoia can occur with repeated high doses of some stimulants over a short period of time and excessive doses can cause severely elevated body temperature and cardiac arrhythmias. Heart failure or seizures can be deadly results of stimulant abuse. Stimulants, like other prescription medications, should not be mixed with other medications unless directed by a physician. Especially dangerous is combining stimulants with OTC medications containing decongestants. This can lead to dangerously high blood pressure and an irregular heart rate. Common stimulants include dextroamphetamine (Dexedrine and Adderall) and methylphenidate (Ritalin and Concerta).

Drastic Measures to Get Drugs

Simply because a drug can be obtained from reputable physicians for legitimate medical purposes does not diminish the fact that certain prescription medications can be powerfully addictive and dangerous. There are many fraudulent ways to obtain prescription drugs. Physicians may inadvertently contribute to a person's addiction by giving that person the benefit of the doubt when he presents a complaint of severe pain that nothing but a narcotic pain reliever will help. That same person may visit other physicians, urgent care clinics, and emergency rooms with similar stories and collect a considerable store of prescription drugs.

Other drastic measures someone might take to obtain prescription drugs are forging prescriptions, stealing or photocopying prescription pads, counterfeiting prescriptions, posing as a physician or office staff when calling a pharmacy ordering a prescription, stealing from doctors' offices, pharmacies, or individuals, buying prescription drugs on the streets, or dealing with dishonest medical personnel.

Federal and state agencies are beginning to work together and are enacting stronger legislation to help curb the illicit use and illegal procurement of prescription drugs. Pharmacists are required to keep more detailed records of all prescriptions they dispense. Patients who require prescription drugs are monitored through computerized records. Tamper-resistant prescription pads or electronically transmitted prescriptions are now being used. Internet pharmacies and their employees as well as dishonest physicians and health care workers are being targeted for investigation and prosecution if appropriate.

 Fact

> You might see advertisements for purchasing prescription medications from foreign countries. The appeal for many is to get needed medications inexpensively. For an addict, it is a source for her addictive substance. However, this is illegal and violates the Federal Food, Drug, and Cosmetic Act. These drugs are not FDA approved and may be of substandard quality.

Talking to a Loved One about His or Her Problem

Having a friend or loved one who is addicted to prescription medications can be confusing and frightening. Initially, one might rationalize that the person really needs the medication and once the pain or other medical problem subsides, the problem will go away. In reality, this is unlikely and it's better to face the problem truthfully.

Timing is important in talking with an addicted person. If the addicted person is not sober at the time of the conversation, she may not be able to have a rational conversation. At the right time, open the conversation with reassurances of care and concern, not condemnation. Learn the facts about prescription drug addiction so the conversation is based on accurate information. An addict may feel shame over her addiction or may feel desperate to obtain more of the drug. Both situations are often motivation for the addict to lie and steal. Confront lying and theft with the truth. It is not helpful to enable an addicted person. The addicted person needs help and treatment and may not be able to recognize the depth of his addiction on his own. Compassion for a painful situation is necessary and may provide the impetus for the addict to trust someone for help. Even though talking with a friend or loved one will hopefully motivate him to get treatment, precautions to protect oneself may be necessary. Lock up prescription medications, money, and valuables. Monitor credit card bills to make sure the cards haven't been used for online prescription drug purchases.

 Alert

> The "shadow market" is a complex system of illicit distribution of prescription drugs. Unscrupulous middlemen divert drugs from legitimate pharmaceutical companies and sell them illegally at huge markups in price. Counterfeiters produce copies of popular, expensive drugs and sell them to unsuspecting pharmacies and patients. Some diverted drugs are diluted before being sold to increase profits.

If medications are left over after an illness has been treated, flush the remainder down the toilet or take it to a pharmacist for proper and safe disposal. Persistently offering to help and letting the addicted person know that you care and are available when he is ready to receive treatment are important.

Getting Help

The good news is that prescription drug addiction can be effectively treated. However, there isn't any one treatment that is effective for all prescription drug addictions. Treatment will be dependent on the type of drug used, the length of time the person has been addicted, and the characteristics of the individual herself. Because of the severity of withdrawal symptoms with many prescription drugs, detoxification under medical supervision is often necessary for a safe start to recovery. Some prescription drug addictions can be treated medically. For example, opiate addiction can be treated with naltrexone, methadone, and buprenorphine. Naltrexone blocks the effects of opiates and is used to treat conditions of opiate overdose as well as the addiction itself. Methadone is a synthetic opiate that blocks the effects of opiates, treats withdrawal symptoms, and helps curb cravings. Buprenorphine was approved by the FDA in 2002. It is also an opiate, but in low doses can be used effectively to discontinue addictive use without experiencing withdrawal symptoms. Treatment for CNS depressant addiction must be medically supervised. Dosages must be reduced gradually to avoid potentially life-threatening withdrawal symptoms.

Essential

Don't assume that prescription drug addiction can't happen to you or someone you care about. An estimated 20 percent of the American population has acknowledged using prescription drugs for nonmedical purposes at some point in their lives.

At this time, there are no approved medical treatments for stimulant addiction. As with other addictions, behavioral and/or cognitive-behavioral therapies have been demonstrated to be effective. Recovery support groups such as Narcotics Anonymous (NA) are also helpful. Therapy and support groups for family members may also be beneficial. Addictions are not a solitary affliction. They affect the lives of many who care for the addicted person. The stronger the support system, the more successful it is in helping the addict gain strength for recovery.

CHAPTER 9

Food Addiction

FOOD ADDICTION IS one of the most frustrating of all the addictions. People have to eat to live, so complete abstinence is just not an option. An alcoholic can stay away from people who drink and avoid bars, but where can a food addict go to avoid food and people who eat? The obvious answer is nowhere. Triggers often can't be avoided and the food addict typically faces a lifetime battle for health.

When Food Becomes More than Nutrition

Aren't all people born with sensations of hunger? Aren't such sensations a necessary part of human survival? Of course. Letting a person know he is hungry is the job of the hypothalamus. The hypothalamus is the part of the brain that monitors glucose levels in the blood. Glucose is a form of sugar, and changes in blood levels of glucose regulate your feelings of hunger.

Food is certainly about more than just fulfilling the hunger urge. Vitamins, minerals, protein, carbohydrates, and other nutrients in the proper proportions are necessary for optimal functioning of your body. In fact, the U.S. Department of Agriculture has devised a food pyramid as a handy guideline to healthy eating. The food pyramid helps you determine the appropriate amounts of fruits, vegetables, dairy products, proteins, and carbohydrates necessary for optimal health. When the amount of food you eat exceeds these guidelines by large amounts (or barely meets these guidelines) it's a sign that you are using food for more than just nutrition for your body.

While it is still a topic for debate, more and more evidence suggests that foods can be addictive. Similar behaviors noted between overeating and substance abuse include compulsive use in spite of negative consequences, cravings, denial, obsessive thoughts about the substance, increased usage as time goes on, guilt with excessive use, and relapse.

Alert

> Individuals with food addictions are at risk for developing binge-eating disorder. Up to 4 percent of the U.S. population has binge-eating disorder. Girls and women are more likely to develop this condition than boys and men.

Signs of Food Addiction

How does a person know if she has a food addiction? There are signs that point to possible trouble in this area. The following questions may help someone determine whether she is a food addict:

- Do you use foods to change your mood?
- Is food or drink necessary for you to enjoy a social situation?
- Do you eat moderately in front of others, but gorge in private?
- Do you go for hours without eating and then clean out the refrigerator at night?
- Is a meal incomplete without dessert?

Denial, of course, is as much a problem with food addiction as with any other addictive substance or behavior. It is hard for anyone to acknowledge that he may have no control over his eating behaviors.

Behavioral Contributions to Food Addiction

Behaviors are learned responses to stimuli. That sounds very clinical, but basically, a person learns to behave in ways that are effective in getting things she wants. How does this work with food addictions? If someone is anxious in a social setting, for example, and she experiences a calmer mood after snacking on appetizers, she is likely to repeat this pattern in similar situations in the future.

Question

What emotion most frequently triggers overeating?
Anxiety has been found to be the most common emotion to set off overeating. Food can have a soothing effect that at least temporarily calms one's anxious mood. The problem is that guilt often follows when one realizes how much food has been used to self-medicate. It can become a vicious cycle in which a food addict feels hopelessly trapped.

Many people use food to distract themselves from difficult emotions such as sadness, loneliness, tiredness, anxiety, and anger. This is particularly true if a person has difficulty talking about his feelings. If an overweight person has been teased a lot, then behaviorally it reinforces the feeling that he should keep things to himself as much as possible. After all, when something is emotionally soothing or comforting, it is logical to behave in ways that will keep it working. Family members are theoretically safe people to talk with about things that are troubling, but if there are problems in family relationships, that may not feel like an option. As a behavioral means of dealing with troubling emotions, food is often readily available and can appear very attractive.

The Abuse Connection

From a behavioral perspective, one can see how sexual abuse and eating disorders may be connected. When someone has been sexually violated, extra poundage to make oneself unattractive may feel like protection to prevent a recurrence of the abuse. Additionally, the chemical soothing stimulated by eating sugars, fats, and refined carbohydrates may be a welcome relief from the painful emotions a sexual abuse victim experiences on a regular basis. The possible health hazards from becoming obese may seem worth the risk to someone whose body has been dealt a cruel blow by sexual abuse.

Alert

The connection between sexual abuse and eating disorders is complex. Childhood sexual abuse is a significant risk factor for eating disorders when combined with psychological problems such as anxiety, depression, and a condition known as alexithymia. Alexithymia is being emotionally disconnected from life experiences.

If someone has been a victim of sexual abuse and food addiction has become a way of coping, professional help will be necessary for recovery from both disorders. The combination of sexual abuse and food addiction is typically too complex for someone to manage alone.

Societal Pressure

Social approval is huge in America. The pressures to be thin, to have the "perfect body," to be sexy, and to look young can lead one to behave in unhealthy ways with food. Some individuals, primarily women, may become addicted to withholding food (anorexia) to gain social approval. If that doesn't work and a person just can't get the perceived "cover girl image" she wants, she may binge-eat to soothe her wounded feelings. (Binge eating is defined as eating considerably more food than most other people would eat under similar circumstances.) Make no mistake about it, social pressure is very hard to resist for many people.

Someone with a food addiction is not necessarily overweight. As with other substances of abuse and addiction, a person may use according to different patterns. Some may eat addictive foods daily, on weekends, only on special occasions, specifically during periods of emotional distress, and so forth. A person may save calories to maintain a certain weight by eating only the food he finds addictive, ignoring foods that don't satisfy the cravings. Thus, a food addict may fall anywhere on the weight continuum, although it is more likely that he finds himself overweight.

Essential

Social factors that contribute to the rise of eating disorders include placing high value on the "perfect body," a very narrow definition of beauty, and the tendency to assess people based on their physical appearance rather than their inner strengths. Courage is required to resist this kind of pressure.

Are All Foods Addictive?

Addiction to broccoli, for example, is highly unlikely. Unless, of course, it's covered with butter and cheese. The neurotransmitter theory is applicable once again. Remember that serotonin's function is to promote a sense of peace and well-being, decrease anxiety, and bring about an upbeat mood. Serotonin is also involved in eating behavior and provides one of the signals that tells the body to stop eating when it's had enough. If a person is low on serotonin, that person might eat a whole coconut cream pie without getting a "Stop, you've gone too far!" message. It has long been noted that an individual with a food addiction may very well have a malfunction in her serotonin system. This can get complicated, but basically, carbohydrates, especially refined carbohydrates such as white sugar and white flour, trigger the release of serotonin.

Additionally, tryptophan, an amino acid and a natural precursor to the release of serotonin, is necessary for serotonin to be made available at the nerve ending site. This system of serotonin production through the precursor action of tryptophan and certain foods is involved in food addiction. Tryptophan is found naturally in turkey and milk. One example of a food that combines sugars with the tryptophan found in milk is, of course, ice cream. Ice cream is often a temptation that is hard for a food addict to resist.

 ## Question

What foods tend to trigger real cravings?
The three basic food types that people most often crave are fat, salt, and sugar. This fact is taken advantage of in the snack aisles in grocery stores and convenience food marts. Those aisles are loaded with soda, chips, cookies, and candy, not celery sticks, carrots, and apples.

The Power of Sugar

Sugar affects much more than just your weight. The following degenerative diseases are directly or indirectly caused by regular sugar consumption: hypoglycemia, chronic constipation, intestinal gas, asthma, osteoporosis, obesity, tooth decay, diabetes, chronic stomach upset, arthritis, headaches, heart disease, chronic Candida infections, and inflammatory bowel disease. Individuals with a sugar addiction experience withdrawal symptoms when cut off from refined sugars, including anxiety, irritability, anger, restlessness, difficulty sleeping, and feelings of being overwhelmed. You will likely recognize that many of these symptoms of withdrawal are similar to other addictive substances already discussed.

Increased opiate (endorphin) and dopamine responses seem to be implicated in the dependent reaction of the body to sugar. Again, this is quite similar to the body's response to other substances of addiction. The pleasure pathway is also at work with sugar.

Not Chocolate, Too!

Is chocolate really addictive? There is some evidence that it may be. All commercially made chocolate products contain significant amounts of sugar. However, the addictive nature of chocolate goes beyond the sugar ingredient alone. Chocolate is also known to stimulate the release of endorphins. Endorphins are hormones found naturally in our bodies and provide us with feelings of pleasure and well-being. Chocolate also contains tryptophan. Tryptophan, the amino acid that stimulates the release of serotonin in the brain, can also produce feelings of elation.

 Fact

According to the United States Department of Agriculture (USDA), the average American consumes twenty teaspoons of additive sugar daily. This is over and above sugar that is naturally occurring in foods. The USDA's recommendation is that an individual consume no more than ten additional teaspoons of sugar daily. These excessive amounts of sugar are difficult for the body to handle and take a toll on one's health.

The premenstrual cravings for chocolate that some women experience may be related to a deficiency in magnesium that can contribute to premenstrual tension. Pregnant women experiencing mild anemia may benefit from chocolate's iron content. In addition, cocoa beans contain flavonoids, a natural antioxidant. These flavonoids also work to limit plaque buildup in our blood vessels by limiting the oxidation of cholesterol. Chocolate increases nitric oxide levels, which helps to relax the inner wall of our blood vessels and thus improves circulation. As it turns out, there are actually many potential benefits to chocolate as well as the addictive qualities. Moderation is the key.

The Lure of the Drive-Through Window

It is very easy to feed one's food addiction. It's legal, it's convenient, and compared to other addictive substances, it's relatively inexpensive. Anyone who has waited in line at a drive-through window at mealtime knows there's lots of company in the craving for refined carbohydrates, sugars, and fats.

 Alert

McDonald's only offered the small size of French fries in the 1950s. Now there are three sizes available, including the super-size serving. Portion sizes of cookies, pasta, crackers, and soda found in restaurants and grocery stores are also much larger than they used to be and significantly larger than portions recommended by the U.S. Department of Agriculture.

People experience so much pressure these days to work harder and for longer hours that fast food may often seem unavoidable for those who want something to eat. Grabbing food at the drive-through window on the way to the office in order to eat and work simultaneously is a common phenomenon. Taking an hour off for a leisurely, healthy lunch of broiled fish and vegetables is not always encouraged or allowed. It's not hard for someone to rationalize that potentially addictive foods are better than skipping meals. Certainly many fast-food chains and convenience stores now offer salads and other "healthier" choices and a person could prepare healthy foods at home to bring, but for a food addict, it's often hard to make those selections when so many of the foods he craves are also on the menu.

Is there any way to combat the lure of fast food that may trigger food addiction without sacrificing convenience? Yes, but it takes planning and being purposeful about choices. Many fast-food restaurants have responded to the cry for healthier foods. Salads, baked potatoes, chili, and fruit cups now often are on the menu. Sandwiches can be ordered with whole-wheat bread and grilled meat. Don't hesitate to make special requests such as eliminating sauces on the sandwiches. Fast-food restaurants are happy to comply with these requests in exchange for repeat customers. Bottled water, milk, and juices are healthier options available instead of the traditional soda.

 Fact

Obesity-related deaths are equivalent to the number of deaths caused by alcohol and tobacco products. If the prevalence of obesity could be reduced, health costs in the United States would be cut by $100 billion to $150 billion per year. This would theoretically reduce the nation's total healthcare budget by 18.7 percent.

If the cravings for French fries, shakes, and burgers seem too strong to resist, take a friend with you through the drive-through. Let your friend know in advance about your struggle and what your plan is for ordering. Sharing the problem with a friend who can be supportive and provide some accountability may mean that convenience doesn't have to be sacrificed in order to maintain abstinence from problem foods.

Talking to a Loved One about His or Her Problem

Talking to someone about his food problems can be difficult. It may be easy to see the problem, but no one wants to bring the subject out into the open. If you really care, take a deep breath and let your friend or loved one know you care enough to take the risk to talk. First, make sure you have your facts straight about food addiction. Do some homework and read up on the subject. Making observations can be less threatening than direct confrontation. For example,

"I've noticed how you sometimes eat a whole package of cookies at a time and then you just seem droopy afterward. I'm concerned."

 Alert

Eating disorders are more widespread than one might think. According to Student Services at Brown University, as many as one in three college women struggle with an eating disorder before graduating from college. Stressors such as school, career, and relationship problems are often cited as triggers that may initiate an eating disorder or exacerbate an existing one.

Genuine compliments about attributes other than appearance may help the food addict to realize she is more than the food she eats. A personal sense of value may translate into "I'm worth addressing this food problem." Express concern and then listen without judgment or condemnation. It is more than likely that the person with a food addiction has spent considerable time already condemning herself. It is never helpful to continually monitor what the food addict is eating. Offer to help, but don't give unsolicited advice. Such advice often puts the food addict in a position where she feels like a "naughty child" instead of an adult who needs to take responsibility for her problem.

 Question

When should someone with a food addiction seek professional treatment?
When life revolves around food and it's difficult to enjoy normal life activities, it's time to seek help. If the fear and anxiety of being discovered binge-eating, hoarding food, or overspending on food controls your life, it's time to get help. If managing food seems out of your control, it's time to get help.

Be a positive role model without communicating condemnation. Offer to exercise with a person at his level, or invite him over to cook a healthy meal together. Take the time to find out the food addict's trigger foods so those are definitely NOT on the menu. Social support can be very helpful, as food addiction is often a disorder developed in secrecy.

Treatment Options

Like other addictions, treatment for food addiction has to target multiple factors to be effective. Physiological, psychological, emotional, social, and spiritual factors are all involved in the picture of food addiction. Symptoms of the food addiction will determine the level and type of care needed to help with recovery. If a person is having serious medical complications resulting from the food addiction, she may require inpatient hospitalization to stabilize her health condition. Physiological issues need to be evaluated by a qualified physician, preferably a physician trained in treating eating disorders.

 Fact

> There is no medication approved by the Food and Drug Administration specifically for treating binge-eating disorder. Some medications that studies have claimed are helpful include a class of antidepressants called selective serotonin reuptake inhibitors (SSRIs), and an antiseizure medication, Topamax.

Although a person with a food addiction might wish for a magic pill to remove the cravings and alleviate the uncomfortable withdrawal symptoms, it doesn't yet exist. However, pharmacological treatment is an area of intense research.

Treatments that focus on changes in behavior are the most effective and accessible to treat food addiction. For people who are medically stable, options to treat food addiction include residential treatment, partial hospitalization treatment, and outpatient treatment with a qualified therapist. Behavioral weight-loss programs may help. However, the primary focus of these programs is on weight loss and not the food addiction per se.

Some people successfully treat their food addictions themselves through self-help programs. One only has to look at the grocery store checkout aisle to see countless magazine articles on weight loss. Some are very helpful and others are clearly fad diets that may not be healthy. A person must use good judgment and do his own research before embarking on one of these plans. Bookstores carry many volumes of the latest how-to instructions for treating eating disorders, including food addiction. Again, this can be an excellent source of help and information, but one must be careful. Consult a professional for advice if in doubt.

Essential

Changing thought patterns about food is equally as important as managing the physical addiction. Self-hatred and low self-esteem lead to a cycle of further overeating and comfort eating. Unless these psychological components are treated, programs of food management are unlikely to be successful.

In treating the behavioral, emotional, and spiritual components of food addiction, twelve-step programs are very popular. Overeaters Anonymous (OA) is well established in helping individuals conquer this addictive behavior. The key is to identify the specific foods that trigger the addictive behavior and to abstain from only those foods. Remember, most likely that's going to be sugar and refined carbohydrates. OA sponsors help with the process and provide support along with a group of peers who are experiencing similar battles. As with treating other addictions, relapses may occur and it may take several attempts before successful recovery is achieved. Don't let this be discouraging! Stay the course and recovery can be enjoyed.

CHAPTER 10

Behavioral Addictions

IT CONTINUES TO be controversial to consider behaviors as addictions. There are those who believe that referring to a behavior such as shopping/spending, exercise, television, and so forth as an addiction is only an excuse for being irresponsible. However, there is more and more evidence to suggest that certain behaviors do exhibit characteristics that qualify them to be included as addictions. Both biological and environmental influences have been discovered that help explain out-of-control, impulsive behaviors.

When Does a Hobby Become an Addiction?

Generally, hobbies or special interests are seen as positive outlets to release stress from a busy schedule or to broaden our connection with friends and family. The always-positive nature of these interests is now coming into question. During the 1980s, the psychiatric community began to consider that some interests when taken to extremes might qualify as addictions. Shopping, exercise, television, games, and so forth were heard in conjunction with addiction (e.g., shopping addiction, exercise addiction).

Although these behaviors are harmless pastimes or healthy pursuits for many, there are signs that indicate you've crossed the line into addiction:

- You put the behavior above being with family and friends.
- A feeling of euphoria drives you to continually seek the desired behavior.

- Mood swings may become apparent in connection with the behavior.
- You may obsess over the behavior, spending excessive amounts of time planning and engaging in the behavior.
- Expenditures connected with the behavior may damage your credit or deplete financial reserves, even to the point of bankruptcy.
- Tolerance is built up around the behavior. In other words, you will feel the need for more and more of the activity to get the same "high" feeling.
- Your job or schoolwork may suffer because of more time and focus going toward the addictive behavior.

Essential

As with any other type of addiction, engaging in a behavior, hobby, or interest regardless of harmful consequences is a key component that sets addictions apart from just having fun. The fun disappears when debt, legal problems, and fractured relationships take over one's life.

When these signs begin to accumulate in your life, you need help. It may be hard for someone to distinguish between having an exciting hobby and an addiction. Any new interest can seem to take over for a time until the new "wears off." Think of what happens when a child gets a new game for his birthday: for the next week, his parents can hardly get him away from the game to the dinner table. The difference between this and a behavioral addiction is that not only does the new not "wear off," it gets worse and it can seemingly take over a person's life.

Impulsive Behavior Versus Addiction

An important question that has been raised by professionals is whether certain behaviors are addictions or whether they belong in the category of impulse-control disorders. Certainly it is believed that there is overlap between the two.

In order to make a comparison between impulse-control disorders and addictions, one must first understand what impulse-control disorders are. Impulse-control disorders are described as failure to resist impulses, drives, and/or temptations to perform acts that may be harmful to the person or to others. The person will feel a mounting accumulation of tension or arousal prior to engaging in the behavior and will then experience pleasure, gratification, or relief when the behavior is finished. The person may or may not experience guilt or regret afterward. Behaviors that have typically been included in the category of impulse-control disorders are intermittent explosive disorder (a failure to resist aggressive impulses), kleptomania (a failure to resist the impulse to steal), pyromania (fire setting for pleasure or relief of tension), pathological gambling, and trichotillomania (pulling out of one's own hair). Compulsive shopping, compulsive computer use, and compulsive sexual behaviors have been proposed as additional impulse-control disorders. More details of these behaviors will be discussed later. Although there may be an obsessive quality to these behaviors, they are not considered to be obsessive-compulsive disorder (OCD) and OCD is not included in the category of impulse-control disorders or addictions.

 Alert

There is a very high co-occurrence between addictive behaviors and other mental health disorders. Mood disorders, anxiety disorders, psychotic disorders, and antisocial personality disorder are commonly seen in individuals struggling with addictive behaviors. One possible and plausible explanation is that addictive behaviors may initially be used inappropriately to relieve symptoms of other mental health problems.

At this time, there are no definitive answers as to whether impulse-control disorders and addictions are distinctly different or two names for the same problem. Research is only beginning to focus on understanding these behaviors in more depth. There are significant indications that biology and genetics as well as environmental factors are involved in these disorders. Technology is now available to study these areas, and it will be exciting to see what knowledge will be gained from ongoing research. Common links between addictions and impulse-control disorders clearly exist. The impulsive nature of the behaviors, poor decision-making abilities, and the failure to accurately evaluate risks versus rewards are evident in both addictive and impulse-control disorders.

Shopping/Spending Addiction

Shopping is a necessary part of life. One shops for food, clothing, cars, homes, or anything consumable in the economic world. If shopping is necessary, how can it also be an addiction? The answer is the same as with other addictions. When a behavior such as shopping becomes an addiction, the motivation for the behavior, the feelings connected with the behavior, the biological effects of the behavior, and the consequences of the behavior are different.

 Fact

Compulsive buying, otherwise known as oniomania, is estimated to occur in 2 to 8 percent of the American population, although it has been observed to occur worldwide in any country with a market-based economy. Approximately 90 percent of those affected are women. This disorder typically begins to appear in the late teens or early twenties.

Initially, the motivation for shopping may seem completely justifiable. A person *needs* groceries, clothing, personal items, even items for entertainment. With a shopping addiction, the rationalization of needing things often covers emotional pain, emptiness, and/or depression. In fact, as with other behavioral addictions, shopping/ spending addictions are commonly seen simultaneously with mood and anxiety disorders, eating disorders, personality disorders, and substance addictions. There is also some research evidence that a genetic component is involved. Compulsive buying happens significantly more often with an individual who also has first-degree relatives with similar symptoms. There is also evidence that, once again, the dopamine pleasure circuit may be involved. The feeling of pleasure triggered in the brain when a person engages in his spending addiction reinforces his desire to do it again. So what are some specific signs of shopping/spending addiction? Here are some of the key things to watch for:

- You consistently spend over your budget and beyond what your income can support.
- You tend to hide the majority of your purchases for fear of criticism.
- You may have multiple secret credit card accounts.
- You may feel shame, guilt, and embarrassment after a spending spree.
- Shopping/spending is motivated by wanting to feel better when depressed or anxious.
- You may begin lying about the amount of money you spent or the items you bought.
- Excessive amounts of items may be purchased. For example, you might legitimately need a pair of shoes, but buy ten pairs instead of the one pair needed.
- Relationships may be damaged through arguments over spending and debt.
- You think obsessively about money and the next shopping outing.

Another characteristic common to shopping/spending addiction is having many items purchased that are never used. In fact, a shopping addict will often have racks of clothes in her closet with the price tags still on them. She may not even remember purchasing the majority of these items. Guilt may motivate a person to return items she has purchased to get her money back. Although this may avoid the accumulation of debt, going back to the store can trigger the temptation to spend again, thus setting up a vicious cycle.

Essential

Shopping/spending addiction is a chronic disorder. It is much more than "going overboard" buying too many presents over the holidays. This is a very serious addiction that can easily lead to financial ruin and broken relationships if not treated. Professional help may be necessary and you should not hesitate to access outside resources.

Denial and rationalization concerning the problem of spending is just as prevalent as with other addictions. Relationships often suffer as friends aren't repaid, collection agencies begin calling the house, necessary family bills can't be paid, extra jobs need to be taken on to pay debt, and other family members do without because of the shopping addict's out-of-control use of resources. A person may begin to isolate herself from the family as shopping expeditions take up more and more of her time. Lying and deception about spending will break trust with the addict's family and friends. Bankruptcy and ruined credit ratings are not unusual consequences for a shopping/spending addict.

Fairly recent complications in the problem of shopping/spending addiction are the proliferation of "infomercials" and television channels devoted to shopping and the rise of Internet shopping. These venues for shopping are deadly for a shopping addict. They are convenient, one never has to leave the comfort of his home to engage in his addiction, and they take credit cards without a hassle. Often, these venues will offer enticing "deals" that are only offered for a limited time or only online. Even staying at home may not be safe any longer for the shopping/spending addict who is trying to resist her urges to spend. Can anything be done to help? Yes! Here are some suggestions to start a person on the road to recovery.

- Destroy all credit cards and commit to paying for items with cash only.
- When shopping for necessary items, make a list prior to shopping and stick to it.
- Don't shop alone—take a friend or family member.
- Avoid discount warehouses where one is encouraged to buy in volume.
- "Window shop" after stores are closed or leave all money at home.

While there is no standard treatment for shopping/spending addiction, several treatment interventions have been found helpful. Taking advantage of financial counseling or debt counseling can help one learn how to wisely manage money and/or repay debt. Individual and group psychotherapy can help one deal with the addiction as well as other mental health problems that may be occurring simultaneously.

 Question

Is there medical treatment for shopping/spending addiction?

Fluvoxamine (Luvox) and other selective serotonin reuptake inhibitors (SSRIs) have been used to treat the obsessive quality of spending addiction. Although medical treatment for this disorder is still in the early research stages, hope is more realistic than ever before.

Exercise Addiction

With more and more attention given to the need for healthier lifestyles, what could possibly be wrong with exercise? The answer is nothing, when used as an adjunct to a balanced plan for developing and maintaining good health and there are no prohibiting medical factors. However, when exercise takes over a person's life, the potential for addiction is there.

 Fact

Exercise addiction is highly correlated with eating disorders. Exercise addiction typically begins with a desire to lose weight. It is unclear at this time whether exercise addiction is a secondary component of eating disorders or if it is a completely separate disorder. Certainly not all individuals with eating disorders develop an exercise addiction, which further complicates this diagnostic dilemma.

Two diagnostic criteria have been identified as necessary for someone to have exercise addiction. There must be impaired functioning in at least two of these areas: psychological, social, occupational, physical, and behavioral. Secondly, as with other addictions, withdrawal symptoms appear when the behavior is stopped. Within twenty-four to thirty-six hours of no exercise, the withdrawal symptoms of anxiety, irritability, nervousness, and guilt may be expected to appear. It is strongly suspected that exercise addiction may produce changes in the brain. A study done with mice demonstrated that when these mice were denied exercise after an intense run, they were found through brain scans to have increased levels of brain activity in sixteen out of twenty-five brain regions. The affected areas of the brain were the same as those connected to cocaine, morphine, alcohol, or nicotine withdrawal. It is known that in humans, vigorous exercise triggers the release of endorphins in the brain. Remember that endorphins are the body's natural opiates and they serve to relieve pain and act as a natural tranquilizer, both of which are powerful reinforcers for exercise.

How do you know if you are addicted to exercise? There are some definite signs to watch for, including:

- You may develop a regularly scheduled pattern of exercise that you feel you must follow to avoid anxiety.
- Exercise takes priority over all other activities.
- You notice an increased tolerance to exercise, beyond what would be typically expected.
- You experience withdrawal symptoms (such as those already described) following the discontinuation of exercise. When exercise is resumed, you feel intense relief.
- You may become aware of a compulsive drive to exercise or others around you may note this and remark on it to you.
- You engage in exercise in spite of injuries or physical deterioration.

It is also concerning when a person significantly increases his exercise time to multiple hours per day or seems to always want to exercise alone. For an exercise addict, the exercise may begin to interfere with healthy social interactions. He may decline going to a party with friends or may forgo family activities in favor of exercise. Work productivity or schoolwork may suffer as the person focuses the majority of his attention on his exercise regimen.

Alert

A healthy exercise routine will build muscle, improve cardiac functioning, and help a person maintain an appropriate weight for her frame, among other things. An exercise addiction often leads to muscle deterioration, physical weakness, exacerbation of injuries that are not given time to heal, and an unhealthy, low body weight. The addict herself may or may not recognize these problems.

Exercise addiction is similar to food addictions in that both exercise and food are essential to life. Therefore, abstinence is not the answer. What can help? A person who is addicted to exercise will need help from knowledgeable individuals. She might join a gym and work out under the supervision of a professional trainer familiar with her problem. Working out in a class with other people can be motivating as well as beneficial in establishing a healthy pattern of exercise. Certainly a physical examination by one's doctor will provide an objective evaluation of whether an exercise program is helping or harming one's body. If there is an associated eating disorder present, professional help is absolutely necessary for recovery. That might be individual and/or group therapy, inpatient or partial hospitalization treatment, or residential treatment, depending on the severity of the disorder.

Other Behavioral Addictions

While it may seem now that anything and everything can be addictive, one must remember the basic criteria for addictions that were described in Chapter 2. Certainly anything can be taken to excess, but that alone doesn't make a substance or a behavior addictive. With that in mind, there are other behaviors that are now thought to have the potential for addiction.

Work Addiction

Work addiction, otherwise known as workaholism, has yet to be adequately researched. Therefore, there is not a clear or complete understanding of how this disorder affects a person psychologically and physiologically.

A workaholic may suffer depression, anxiety, anger, high blood pressure, and a weakened immune system resulting from the chronic stress he experiences. There are typically three stages of workaholism. In the early stage, the person is constantly busy and can't say no to extra work. He will put in many extra hours without pay and feels stressed at the thought of taking time off. The middle stage of workaholism finds the person becoming emotionally more attached to his work than to family, friends, or other interests. He may begin to notice physical problems such as insomnia or weight loss as he invests more of himself in his work. In the final stage, the workaholic will begin to experience more serious physical, emotional, and social problems. He may develop chronic headaches, high blood pressure, ulcers, depression, anxiety, and so forth.

Like other addictions, work addiction often develops as an attempt to cope with emotional pain or low self-esteem. The adrenaline rush one feels as a result of successfully meeting a demanding deadline is very reinforcing. Unlike most other addictions, which often thrive in secrecy, work addiction derives much of its reinforcement from public praise, promotions, and bonuses.

Essential

Constant work, whether physical or sedentary, leads to chronic stress. Workaholics have significantly more physical and mental health problems than nonworkaholics do. According to Bryan E. Robinson in his book, *Chained to the Desk: A Guidebook for Workaholics, Their Partners and Children, and the Clinicians Who Treat* Them, the health-related costs of workaholism may be as much as $150 billion per year.

Work addiction is a progressive disorder that worsens with time. A solid work ethic is commendable, but the following signs may indicate that someone is slipping into work addiction.

- Relationships with family and friends become strained or broken.
- Health problems develop and progress.
- A work addict often becomes obsessed with control and power. She may become rigid and inflexible in her work habits.

- Productivity at work eventually suffers. As the work addict takes on more to do, she is less able to organize and utilize coworkers to help with the load. Work quality diminishes.
- Frustration mounts and the work addict reaches the place where no amount of work or success is enough to fulfill her need for emotional peace and security.

Developing balance in one's life is the key to recovery. A person may not be able to achieve this balance without help and guidance. A physician's care will be necessary to manage the physical complications of work addiction. Under the physician's supervision, the work addict will need to cultivate healthy eating and exercise regimes. Getting adequate rest and nurturing one's spiritual health will also be helpful. Social interaction is important. For the work addict, it may take intentional planning to balance his social life with his work life. Personal health and well-being along with satisfying family relationships will give the addict the personal peace he's been craving. At work, the addict may benefit from a personal coach who can help with organization, setting appropriate goals, pacing the work, and establishing healthy productive relationships with coworkers. Workaholics Anonymous is a twelve-step program that can also provide support for the work addict.

 Fact

Addictive compulsive shoplifters make up approximately 75 percent of individuals caught stealing. Kleptomania is an impulse-control disorder and is relatively rare, occurring in fewer than 5 percent of identified shoplifters.

Shoplifting Addiction

An addiction to shoplifting is more common than one might think. In fact, it has been estimated by the National Association for

Shoplifting Prevention that one out of eleven individuals in the United States has engaged in shoplifting.

Someone who is addicted to shoplifting cares very little about what he steals. A shoplifting addict steals because he enjoys a sense of euphoria from the act of stealing without being caught. A person who is addicted to shoplifting often throws the items away or gives them to friends or family members. It is common for someone with a shoplifting addiction to also have other addictions, such as gambling, food, or substance addictions. He may also suffer from a co-occurring mental health problem. A shoplifting addiction is very different from theft. Ordinary theft may be planned or impulsive. Theft is deliberate and is motivated by the usefulness or monetary value of the item stolen. The following list contains indications that a person's shoplifting may be addictive:

- She may lose time from work, school, or family activities because of the shoplifting.
- Shoplifting may be creating problems in relationships.
- She will feel a "rush" or sense of euphoria after shoplifting.
- Shoplifting may be motivated by emotional upsets, frustrations, or arguments and is done to soothe herself.
- Shoplifting is typically a secret activity, even from those closest to the shoplifter.
- She will continue the activity in spite of the legal consequences, a damaged reputation, or broken relationships. In fact, the urge to shoplift will increase, as it is a progressive disorder.
- She will be consumed with thinking about it, planning for it, and engaging in the activity.

As with many other addictive disorders, a twelve-step group has been developed specific to the problem of shoplifting. Cleptomaniacs and Shoplifters Anonymous (CASA) is a support group committed to using the twelve-step approach to helping a shoplifting addict achieve recovery. Individual psychotherapy may be helpful in treating underlying contributing factors that promote the addiction. If there are coexisting mental health problems, they will need to be treated by a professional mental health care provider. This will help with recovery from shoplifting addiction as well. Multiple problems will need a multidisciplinary approach for effective treatment.

Effects on Family Members

There is no question that behavioral addictions can have devastating effects on one's family members as well as on the addict himself. The sorrow that family members feel over the suffering of their loved one may be compounded with financial consequences of repaying debt or helping fund treatment. Guilt, embarrassment, shame, anxiety, and grief are common and understandable feelings that family members may experience. Then they often experience further guilt when they acknowledge those painful feelings in connection with someone they care about so much.

 Alert

> Behavioral addictions can take family members by surprise. Many addictions that fall into this category, such as exercise addiction, seem like positive healthy outlets in the beginning. This makes it much easier to rationalize, deny, and ignore the problem family members may suspect in their addicted loved one.

Family members also need support, whether that occurs in a therapeutic support group or in individual or family therapy. It is very difficult to know how to set appropriate limits with an addicted loved one while at the same time wanting to be perceived by the addict as supportive. This requires courage and wisdom beyond what one might expect. Fear can be overwhelming. Family members fear what their addicted loved one may have to go through as a result of the addiction. Jail, bankruptcy, divorce, and hospitalization are all realistic possibilities. Family members may not be able to face their fears alone; again, help is needed and one should not hesitate to seek it out.

Talking to a Loved One about His or Her Problem

Gentle, caring, but firm confrontation will be necessary to help a friend or loved one caught in the snare of addiction. Telling the truth with respect, consideration, and care is the most essential element of a confrontation. It is not uncommon for the addicted person to lie about the addiction, deny the problem, rationalize or defend her behavior, and try to avoid this unpleasant subject. However, in time, acknowledging the truth about the problem is the foundation for recovery.

Timing is critical in talking to someone about her addiction. The discussion should be during a time when there will be no interruptions, the addict is "sober," and there are no appointments looming in the immediate future. Think through and plan what you want to say. Once the words are out of your mouth, you can't take them back. As much as possible, make sure the message is honest, straightforward, hopeful, and encouraging. Make it clear that your desire is to provide help and support to the addicted person, not judgment or condemnation.

Seeking Help

It may be hard to know at first what help is needed and what kind of help will be the most effective. A good place to start is to make an appointment with a mental health professional who specializes in working with addictions. Get a thorough assessment of the problem and then use the professional's help to map out an overall treatment plan. The treatment plan may include psychotherapy, support groups, psychiatric management with medications, lifestyle training, and so on. More and more information and research is now available on behavioral addictions. As these types of addictions are taken more seriously in the professional community, there is more funding and interest for research. Hope for recovery is present and growing!

CHAPTER 11

Gambling Addiction

IN RECENT DECADES, gambling has come out into the open and flourished. Mega-casinos have spread from Las Vegas and Atlantic City to cover the country. Gambling is now legal in forty-eight of fifty states. In fact, the United States is now considered the largest national gambling market in the world. Along with this rise in public, legalized gambling comes an escalation in gambling addiction, otherwise known as pathological gambling. While many herald the economic advantages of gambling, the gambling addict who has lost everything on a bet knows the dark side of this behavior.

It's Just Entertainment!

For many, gambling is just entertainment. Casinos may include lavish hotels, celebrity entertainment, and boundless gourmet meals as well as gambling. People may get together with friends for a social evening of poker and snacks or enjoy placing a wager on their favorite ball team while watching Sunday night football together. Vegas Night may be the theme of a charity event involving people having fun playing blackjack or the roulette table while supporting a favorite cause. And who can resist the excitement of calling out "Bingo!" and winning the "pot" of cash?

While entertaining for most, 2 to 4 percent of the population, approximately 2 million people, struggle with the devastating disorder of gambling addiction. Gambling addiction typically begins in the adolescent years for males, and later years for females. However, some studies have suggested that when an individual begins gambling later in life, the progression from social gambling to gambling addiction occurs faster. More research has been conducted on gambling addiction than any other behavioral addiction, but there is still much to learn. What seems apparent so far is that a genetic link and a gender link likely exist in gambling addiction. In other words, an individual is more likely to develop a gambling addiction if he is male and has a first-degree relative who also has a gambling addiction.

 Alert

Many potentially addictive substances and behaviors are more likely to develop into full-blown addictions when use begins in the teen years. Gambling is no exception. In fact, teenagers are three times more likely to become addicted to gambling than adults. This is quite alarming and indicates a great need for early intervention and education regarding gambling.

The Biology of Gambling

It's no surprise to learn that gambling addiction, like other addictions, receives biological reinforcement through the dopamine pleasure pathway. Research is showing that gambling addiction activates the same parts of the brain that substances such as cocaine do. It has also been suggested that pathological gamblers have lower levels of norepinephrine than normal gamblers. Norepinephrine is a neurotransmitter in the brain that imprints information into long-term memory. It is released when a person is experiencing stress or arousal. This is reinforced when someone is aroused by a gambling win and that memory is imprinted on the brain.

Serotonin is yet another neurotransmitter that is implicated in the problem of pathological gambling. Serotonin affects one's moods and behaviors, and it has been well documented that depression often co-occurs with gambling addiction. Other abnormalities have also been discovered in the brains of pathological gamblers. Impairments in the prefrontal cortex of the brain noted in pathological gamblers affect their ability to make sound decisions, to focus and attend, and to control impulses. One can readily understand how these abnormalities in the brain of an addicted gambler can lead to devastating consequences.

 Question

Is pathological gambling an impulse-control disorder or an addiction?

The Diagnostic and Statistical Manual of Mental Disorders, Fourth Edition (DSM-IV) presents diagnostic criteria compiled by the American Psychiatric Association for mental health disorders. In the *DSM-IV*, pathological gambling is described as an impulse-control disorder. However, more up-to-date research is suggesting pathological gambling is more closely related to substance use disorders because of the biological and genetic connections between the two disorders.

The complexities of the brain often lead to multiple mental health problems and addictions, as has been discussed in previous chapters. A person addicted to gambling is also more likely to have other addictions, particularly alcohol, and mental health problems such as mood disorders, adjustment disorders, personality disorders, and anxiety disorders. Alcohol addiction is particularly problematic in combination with gambling addiction, as it leads to further disinhibited behavior and poor decision-making. Keep this in mind when you note that many casinos offer gamblers free alcoholic beverages while they are gambling.

The Phases of Gambling Addiction

Gambling addiction is a progressive disorder. Phases of a gambling addiction are predictable and follow a downward spiral. The winning phase occurs with a big win or a series of smaller wins. The dopamine pleasure pathway is activated and the gambler is unreasonably certain that the winning streak will go on indefinitely. The excitement he feels is heightened with the increasing amounts of his bets. Inevitably, a losing phase follows. The gambler may start gambling alone to hide the losses. He may go into debt and borrow money, and he may begin to experience a downward plunge emotionally with irritability, depression, and restlessness. Lying about gambling activities often begins in this phase and the gambler will feel compelled to gamble more in order to recoup his losses. The desperation phase finds the gambler spending more time and attention to his gambling behavior. It is not uncommon for the gambling addict to now begin financing his gambling with illegal activities. Emotional and psychological problems escalate and more serious consequences ensue such as arrests, divorce, bankruptcy, and so forth.

Fact

Desperation motivates many gambling addicts to commit illegal acts to fund their gambling behavior. One study found that two out of three gambling addicts turned to crime to pay gambling-related debts. Not only does this lead to painful consequences for the gambling addict and her family, it puts an additional burden on our country's legal system.

Finally, the addicted gambler may enter the hopelessness phase. At this point, he sees no way out of his situation. Thoughts of suicide are common. In fact, in this phase of the addiction, approximately 20 percent of gambling addicts will attempt suicide.

Essential

Environmental influences also affect gambling addiction. For example, a person who lives close to a gambling facility is more likely than others to develop a gambling addiction. Someone whose friends regularly gamble will be more readily drawn into problem gambling behavior.

Watch for the Signs

A gambling addict may become involved with the behavior initially for one of two reasons. Some enjoy the euphoric thrill of the risks and action, while others use gambling to help manage emotional or psychological problems. The signs and symptoms of gambling addiction reflect these situations. How does one know if he has a problem with gambling addiction? The following criteria will help evaluate the problem:

- He will be preoccupied with gambling, talking excessively about his wins or making plans for his next gambling outing.
- He will require more and more money to bet to arouse the same level of excitement.
- He will try to control or stop the behavior, but be unable to succeed.
- Withdrawal symptoms such as irritability and restlessness will appear when he tries to stop the behavior.
- He will use gambling to relieve emotional distress or to escape unpleasant life situations.
- His gambling will escalate as he tries to win back lost money.
- He will use lies and deception to cover his gambling addiction.
- He may participate in illegal or criminal acts to fund his gambling.
- He will borrow money from friends and family, even illegal sources, to cover his gambling debts.
- Gambling will dominate his life, taking precedence over family, friends, and career.

As you can see, among other signs, tolerance and withdrawal are as much a part of gambling addiction as other addictions. Gambling addiction is not simply a problem with managing one's entertainment money. It is an uncontrollable obsession that impacts all areas of one's life.

Other behaviors surrounding gambling that may indicate a problem include feeling remorseful or guilty after gambling. Someone may use his paycheck to pay gambling debts instead of the mortgage or phone bill. He may find that he's spent more time gambling than he intended. A gambling addict may find he's losing sleep or can't eat because of preoccupation with gambling. Even though he may have set a monetary limit for himself before going gambling, he finds he overspends until his last dollar is gone. Without a doubt, when gambling reaches the point of addiction, complications will appear. Loss of family and friends, legal problems, financial problems, difficulties with school or one's job, and the development of other addictions or mental health disorders signal a need for professional help.

Gambling Is Good for the Economy, Right?

Apparently, state governments believe this to be true. Gambling is now legal in forty-eight states, the District of Columbia, Puerto Rico, and the U.S. Virgin Islands. Only Hawaii and Utah do not have state-authorized gambling. Forty-one states in this country have state lottery systems, all of which are state-owned monopolies.

 Question

What is a "gray market?"
A "gray market" is an area where the legality of gambling is unclear. In many states, gambling games such as slot machines are located in truck stops, convenience stores, bars, and so forth but the legality of these operations is not clearly defined. Businesses allow gambling in these situations at their own risk.

What does legalized gambling encompass? Bingo is legal in forty-seven states and betting on horse racing, dog racing, and other sports is legal in at least forty-one states. Lotto, keno, and instant lottery games are legal in forty-one states and the District of Columbia. Thirty-three states have some type of casino operations, both commercial and tribal. Tribal casinos are those operated by Native Americans. In 1988, the Indian Gaming Regulatory Act was passed and allows Native American tribes to operate any form of gambling that is legal in the state where the tribe is located. Casinos allow for a wide variety of gambling opportunities such as card games, roulette, and slot machines. With all of this legalized gambling, the question remains, is it beneficial to the economy? On the plus side, it is argued that legalized gambling creates additional jobs with higher incomes, encourages economic gains from the tourism industry, and leads to higher property values in the area. More and more, state governments base a significant part of their budgets on the proceeds from state-operated gambling. While this sounds good, it's not the whole story.

Essential

> The types of gambling that lead most quickly to gambling addiction are those that are fast-paced and immediately reinforcing. Video poker and slot machines are two examples of gambling that can progress to the desperation phase of gambling addiction within a relatively brief period of time.

The social costs of gambling represent the arguments against legalization. Social costs are those costs that are overt or hidden and become a burden to society at large. Nine examples of the social costs of gambling have been identified:

- Crime is very costly to society in terms of apprehension, adjudication, incarceration, and staffing of law enforcement. As many as two-thirds of gambling addicts may resort to crime to fund their addiction.
- It has also been argued that employment costs, in terms of lost productivity and lost employment time, equal or outweigh the benefits of jobs gained in the gambling industry.

- Bankruptcy is another social cost of gambling. Legal costs, debt collection costs, and lawsuits make bankruptcy a very expensive solution to a gambler's money problems.
- Suicide is common among gambling addicts. The emotional costs of suicide cannot begin to be measured. The loss of the person's skills and talents to society as well as his contribution to his family is immense.
- Pathological gamblers are also vulnerable to stress-related illnesses such as cardiovascular diseases, severe headaches, and gastrointestinal disorders.
- Mental health problems such as depression and anxiety are common occurrences in gambling addicts.
- The social costs of health care related to gambling addiction are quite significant. You will recall that gambling addiction is highly correlated with alcohol addiction and other addictions that are also quite expensive to treat.
- Social service costs related to gambling addiction include welfare, costs associated with unemployment, and therapy costs.
- Divorce and broken relationships due to gambling create both emotional and financial costs.

 Fact

Remember, it is not the amount of money won or lost that makes a person a gambling addict. It is not even the impact the gambling addict's behaviors have on society or her family. Gambling becomes an addiction when a person loses control of her gambling behavior and experiences tolerance and withdrawal symptoms when trying to stop.

Of course, with state governments so directly involved in legalized gambling, there are regulatory costs that are passed along to the taxpayer. The families of gambling addicts often bear a huge cost as well.

Costs associated with divorce, separation, child abuse and neglect, and spousal abuse can become astronomical. Finally, there are the costs accrued to family, friends, and employers when the gambling addict takes advantage of them and extracts money under false pretenses.

Internet Gambling

Internet gambling may be more dangerous to the average American than other forms of legalized gambling. A person can sit in the comfort and anonymity of his home and lose thousands of dollars, as well as quality time with his family. In fact, in 2005, approximately 8 million Americans engaged in Internet gambling, playing poker, blackjack, and sports betting to the tune of around $12 billion. Without a doubt, online poker is the most popular Internet gambling game. Internet gambling has become such a problem in this country that the U.S. government has begun to take action to limit its accessibility. In 1961, the Wire Act was passed to prohibit certain types of gambling businesses from operating. This Act has recently been used as grounds for restricting the operation of sports betting websites as well.

In 2006, President George Bush signed into law the Unlawful Internet Gambling Enforcement Act. This law prohibits Americans from using electronic funds transfers, credit cards, and checks to place bets with gambling sites operated by foreign companies. Banks and credit card companies are responsible for enforcing this law. The law does not criminalize Internet gambling. However, it is designed to restrict certain financial transactions, making it more difficult to be involved with Internet gambling.

The Effects on Families Are Not Fun

The gambling addict is not the only one to suffer from this addiction. The effects of gambling addiction can quickly throw a family into crisis. One immediately thinks of the financial impact on families such as debt repayment, bankruptcy, bad credit ratings, and so forth. Related to this, the gambling addict may have lost his job or may be arrested for embezzlement, fraud, or check forgery. Even one's home may be lost and go into foreclosure when the mortgage payments can't be made. Family members may feel they need a second job to save the family financially.

 Question

Who are "casino kids?"

"Casino kids" are the children of gambling addicts who may be left in cars or on sidewalk curbs while their parents are gambling. Children of gambling addicts are frequently neglected or abandoned physically and emotionally by a parent who is caught up in his or her addiction. Abuse is common, and these children are more likely to develop a gambling addiction themselves.

The emotional trauma a family may experience can also be devastating. A family member other than the addict may be the one confronted and harassed by debt collectors and creditors. Dealing with divorce, separation, or being the only parent trying to manage the home front while the gambling addict is gone can feel overwhelming. Families may experience shame, guilt, and embarrassment over their financial circumstances or having their loved one in prison facing serious legal consequences. It will be essential for family members to develop support systems and get professional help to see them through this difficult situation. Only families who are emotionally and mentally healthy will be able to support their loved one trying to recover from gambling addiction.

Confronting the Game

Empathy for the gambling addict will be necessary in order to help. Family members and loved ones affected by the spillover consequences of the gambling addict may justifiably feel hurt and angry.

Nevertheless, remember that gathering accurate information about one's circumstances, being truthful, and developing a comprehensive treatment plan for the family and the gambling addict will be necessary for recovery. Lying and deception are common behaviors of someone in the grip of gambling addiction. The gambling addict needs to be confronted firmly but with compassion. Someone with professional intervention skills may be called on to help if necessary. While making it clear to the gambling addict that you want to support her and help in her recovery, it is also important that she be respectfully told how her addiction has affected those around her. Taking responsibility for one's actions is an important step in recovery and rebuilding one's self-esteem.

Essential

Friends and family members who may have been drawn into the financial problems of the gambling addict need to learn their legal rights and responsibilities. Although one can empathize with the gambling addict, those around him need to protect themselves legally and financially. Hiring a knowledgeable attorney or a financial/debt counselor may be helpful. Don't avoid getting help because of fear or embarrassment.

Treatment Options

Gambling addiction can be successfully treated. In severe cases, such as when a gambling addict is suicidal, stabilization with inpatient treatment will likely be necessary.

Once safety is assured, partial hospitalization programs or outpatient treatment can be effective. Three primary approaches have been found to be beneficial. Psychotherapy, including cognitive-behavioral therapy and group therapy, focuses on identifying irrational, faulty thinking that feeds into the addiction and replacing it with accurate, healthy thoughts. A self-help group such as Gamblers Anonymous is another approach. Again, this is a twelve-step group where the addict gains strength and support from fellow addicts.

 Fact

Certified gambling counselors are professionals who have received a minimum of thirty hours of training specifically designed to treat gambling addiction and the particular problems that gambling addicts face. Once they have completed coursework, they receive a period of additional supervision by an experienced professional before becoming certified by a national or state accrediting organization.

Medications have also brought some relief to individuals suffering from gambling addiction. Selective serotonin reuptake inhibitors (SSRIs) such as clomipramine, citalopram, fluoxetine, and fluvoxamine have been used to treat the impulsiveness associated with gambling addiction. Naltrexone, an opiate antagonist, has also had some success in the treatment of gambling addiction. Lithium has been found to be helpful in treating the more manic symptoms a gambling addict may experience. Of course, co-occurring addictions and mental health problems must also be treated for a full recovery.

CHAPTER 12

Relational Addictions

LOVE AND RELATIONSHIPS are a positive part of human existence that everyone wants and looks forward to with anticipation. Nothing is more exciting than a first date when your eyes meet and a great connection is made. Romantic nights make wonderful memories that can be stored away forever. That is, however, unless you are a person who struggles with love, sex, and relationship addictions. For that person, the frustration of pursuing relationships but never feeling satisfied can become unbearable.

Love Addiction

Healthy love for another person comes out of free choice based on attraction to the other person, one's beliefs about love and commitment, and connection based on mutual interests and goals. Strong feelings and a desire to be with the object of your affection is a normal part of "being in love." But can love possibly become an addiction? Absolutely. Love addiction arises out of environmental, familial, and, once again, chemical upsets in one's life. As with other types of addiction, love addiction has a compulsive component, the development of tolerance, and withdrawal symptoms. Each time a love "high" is achieved, there is a temporary sensation of relief.

The compulsive nature of love addiction is a person's drive to be in a relationship or to be "in love" regardless of whether the relationship is abusive, inappropriate, or destructive in some way. The love addict will feel a sense of panic when a relationship is broken off and she will direct all her energies to either resurrect the broken relationship or immediately find another. Tolerance in love addiction occurs when the addicted person needs more and more from the relationship to feel the same level of excitement as in the beginning. The other person in the relationship is, in a sense, the love addict's "substance." The symptoms of withdrawal from a broken relationship may feel excruciating to the love addict. He may experience sleep disturbances, gastrointestinal upsets, irritability, depression, and anxiety. The craving for the emotional euphoria of love will then drive the addict to find another relationship to pursue.

Essential

Satisfying love relationships promote personal awareness and growth, encouraging the same in others. For someone with a love addiction, relationships and love feelings are used as a way of coping with a life that otherwise feels empty. The intrigue, flirtations, and manipulations involved in love addiction provide a level of excitement missing from ordinary life.

Where does love addiction begin? The roots of love addiction may be found in infancy. The first year of life is when an individual ideally develops a healthy sense of attachment. This occurs when a helpless infant has her needs for love, security, safety, and physical sustenance met by a warm, responsive caretaker. Reactive attachment disorder may develop in the absence of this loving care. Reactive attachment disorder is a disturbed ability to relate socially in most situations and typically shows up as generalized mistrust of people or indiscriminately trusting people. This disorder occurs when an infant's basic emotional needs, physical needs, and/or security needs are not met adequately by the primary caretaker. Reactive attachment disorder may also occur when the existence of multiple caregivers prevents an infant from forming stable attachments.

There are two main subtypes of reactive attachment disorder. An individual suffering from the *inhibited* type of reactive attachment disorder will often remain aloof and uninvolved in social situations. Although she may respond with politeness to friendly overtures, her heart will not be involved in the interaction and she will end the connection as quickly as possible. The likely root of love addiction stems from the *disinhibited* type of reactive attachment disorder. In this situation, a person responds to social situations indiscriminately, or does not show good judgment in selecting people with whom to attach. This individual will try to connect socially with anyone who is willing, whether or not the person is a healthy social choice.

Alert

> Low self-esteem, feelings of inadequacy, and insecurity are common characteristics of a love addict. These qualities put a love addict at risk for submitting herself to abusive, dangerous, and unhealthy relationships in her search for love. A love addict's constant fear of losing her partner may also lead her to engage in desperate measures to retain the attentions of her partner.

Although reactive attachment disorder may result from an abusive, neglectful caretaker, there may also be legitimate reasons why a caretaker is unable to meet the needs of an infant. A caretaker may be physically ill, mentally ill, away in the military, or in other ways unavailable through no personal fault. A child with reactive attachment disorder may grow into an adult who develops a love addiction in an unhealthy attempt to meet this legitimate need for attachment and love. A person may initially develop a love addiction by observing unhealthy relationships within her family system. Parents, extended relatives, or close family friends may have also had a love addiction that served as an example for the addict.

Environmentally, movies, television, and music often represent love addiction as a normal and desirable way of life or as a subject for comedy. For an individual who is susceptible to love addiction, it can be difficult to resist the influence of this unhealthy representation of love perpetrated by the entertainment industry. In addition, what about biological influences on love addiction? The biological chemistry associated with the emotion of love is real, complex, and amazing. Dopamine, norepinephrine, testosterone, phenylethylamine (PEA), and serotonin levels are all associated with the emotion of love. When an individual is feeling romantic, the levels of dopamine increase in the brain's nucleus accumbens and caudate nucleus, and in the ventral tegmental area. This is the region of the brain that forms the reward network that has been discussed in previous chapters. You may recall that this area of the brain is heavily associated with cravings and addictions. It might even be said that increased dopamine levels act like a "love potion." When a person's need for love goes unmet, elevated dopamine levels lead to cravings that intensify with the unavailability of a partner. Additionally, dopamine stimulates an elevation in testosterone levels that increase sexual desire.

 Fact

Levels of phenylethylamine (PEA) increase with feelings of infatuation. Elevations of this brain chemical, which is closely related to amphetamines, lead to feelings of euphoria and excitement when an appealing potential partner comes into view. Chocolate contains PEA and may be why chocolate is often described as an aphrodisiac.

Norepinephrine comes into play by providing energy, feelings of euphoria, and the ability to imprint this wonderful love experience into long-term memory. Remember, having a rewarding experience available in our memory banks serves as a trigger to want more and more. An interesting chemical phenomenon that occurs simultaneously with the rise in dopamine, PEA, norepinephrine, and testosterone is a drop in serotonin levels. The decreased serotonin levels lead to the obsessive qualities associated with love. All else may be forgotten in the pursuit of the love object. When attachment problems, environmental influences, and chemical imbalances converge, one can easily see that love addiction can be a serious and often debilitating disorder. Love addicts are often motivated by fears of change, loss, and abandonment. Taken to the extreme, these fears can result in assaults, suicide, stalking, and even murder. How does a person know if he is a love addict? The following characteristics are commonly seen in a love addict:

- It is very difficult for him to trust in relationships.
- He often has a fear of abandonment and loneliness.
- He may experience intense anger over abuse or the lack of nurturing in childhood.
- He is likely to emotionally attach without taking the time to get to know a person.
- He confuses wants with needs.
- He may behave manipulatively and dependently.
- He will likely become preoccupied with his romantic interests to the point of being unable to concentrate or focus on other activities in his life.
- Emotional emptiness may be present even while he is involved in a relationship.
- Unrealistic qualities and expectations may be attached to the person he is attracted to, along with the belief that only that person can bring him happiness.
- He may spend excessive amounts of money on his romantic interests. Debt and a failure to meet financial obligations may result.

A person with a love addiction will find it very difficult to believe that she is deserving of a healthy love relationship. She is likely to focus more on her partner and pleasing him rather than on developing her own sense of self. In fact, a love addict may continue to worry and obsess about a partner whom she broke off with years ago. Is recovery from love addiction possible? Yes, but as with other addictions, professional help will likely be necessary. Psychotherapy to deal with such issues as attachment disorders, low self-esteem, undeveloped self-identity, lack of social skills, and mood disorders may be quite beneficial to a love addict's recovery. Medication management of mood disorders or other associated mental health problems may also be necessary.

Essential

A love addict will try to regulate his moods through relationships. Depression and anxiety disorders are common. The mood elevations created by a new relationship lead to a false sense of well-being. Professional treatment with therapy and medications may be necessary to help a love addict accurately assess and manage his emotions.

Serial Dating

A serial dater is a person who measures relationships in terms of days, weeks, or at most, a few months. This is someone who is likely dating more than one person at the same time. As with the love addict, a serial dater does not enjoy being alone. If for some reason a dating situation does not go as planned, the serial dater wants an alternative immediately available.

A serial dater may very well have begun dating with the goal of a long-term, satisfying, and committed relationship. Somewhere along the way, the serial dater became more enthralled with the dating than with the commitment. There are several possible explanations for this. A serial dater may have been deeply hurt in a previous relationship and, out of a sense of self-protection, will no longer fully give himself emotionally to another person. She may have a history of childhood sexual abuse and find it difficult to trust a man with commitment. A serial dater may be a perfectionist and so fearful of making a relational mistake that he never takes the risk to pursue a serious connection. Another possibility is someone who has been deeply wounded by parental divorce. Not wanting to go through that experience again, a serial dater prefers short-term companionship with no risk of divorce. Finally, a serial dater may have crossed the line into love and/or sex addiction. In this case, the euphoric and addictive feelings of falling in love over and over again have become out of control.

 Question

What is a "player?"
A "player" is a serial dater, but with a twist. Unlike the serial dater, a player has no intention of pursuing commitment in a relationship. A player may use the illusion of searching for a serious relationship as a means of attracting a partner. In reality, if the partner shows signs of becoming serious, a player will quickly move on.

Sex Addiction

Sex addiction may be somewhat difficult to define simply because the range of what is "normal" sexually is quite broad. Hormonal levels that stimulate sexual desire are different in various individuals. For one person, enjoying sex several times per week is perfectly normal while, for another, once a month might be quite satisfactory.

Sex addiction occurs when a person feels he has lost control over whether or not he engages in sexual behavior. He has likely attempted to stop the compulsive sexual behavior without success. The sex addict will continue to seek out sexual encounters in spite of negative or harmful consequences. Finally, the sex addict obsessively thinks about sex and spends inordinate amounts of time planning the next sexual encounter. The unique patterns of behavior and brain activity found in addictions are true for substance and behavioral addictions alike. Sex addiction encompasses a variety of sexual behaviors including:

- Compulsively masturbating
- Having multiple affairs, either sequential or simultaneous
- Having multiple or anonymous sexual partners and/or one-night stands
- Viewing pornography
- Having unsafe sex
- Engaging in cybersex or phone sex
- Using prostitutes or escort services
- Visiting strip clubs and adult entertainment venues
- Frequenting massage parlors
- Having sexual paraphilias

Alert

Sexually addicted women are at particular risk for unplanned pregnancies, complications from abortions, and violence. Like men, sexually addicted women are also susceptible to sexually transmitted diseases.

More needs to be said about the sexual paraphilias. Sexual paraphilias are recurrent sexually arousing fantasies, sexual urges, or behaviors that are pathological in nature, and frequently illegal. Exhibitionism is the exposure of one's genitals to a stranger, sometimes masturbating as part of the experience. A fetish is the use of a nonliving object, such as women's undergarments, for sexual stimulation. Again, fetishism is frequently associated with masturbation.

Frotteurism is another type of sexual paraphilia and involves touching and rubbing against a nonconsenting person and often occurs in crowded places such as a mall, sports event, or public transportation. Pedophilia is sexual activity with a prepubescent child and is, of course, illegal. Sexual masochism is an act of being humiliated, beaten, bound, and so forth for sexual stimulation and arousal. Sexual sadism involves the infliction of psychological or physical suffering on another for the purpose of sexual excitement. Transvestic fetishism is dressing in clothing of the opposite gender and masturbating while cross-dressed. Finally, voyeurism is the act of watching unsuspecting individuals disrobing or engaging in sexual activity. The voyeur achieves sexual excitement through watching and frequently simultaneously masturbates.

 Fact

Paraphilias are overwhelmingly associated with men. Except for sexual masochism, other paraphilias are a rarity in women. Even in sexual masochism, the ratio is twenty men to one woman in terms of occurrence. However, the accuracy of statistics obtained from Internet sources is questionable because of the ability of respondents to disguise their gender and age.

What causes sex addiction? Psychological factors include fear of intimacy, a negative way of releasing anger, or guilt/shame, which may have stemmed from a history of sexual abuse, familial sexual secrets, or observing the sexual activity of one's parents. Sexually addictive behavior can also be a means of managing stress or numbing emotional pain. Environmental factors may include watching pornography or sexually explicit movies, listening to erotic music lyrics, or being influenced by friends involved in sex addictions.

Biologically, all of the chemistry described in love addiction applies here. Additionally, the desire for sexual release is associated with rising levels of testosterone in both sexes. Interesting to note, testosterone is highest in men early in the morning and in women around ovulation. Testosterone levels fall with the experience of sexual release and then build again to motivate further sexual activity. The brain literally goes wild during an orgasm. The vagus nerves, the reticular formation, basal ganglia, anterior insular cortex, amygdala, cerebellum, and hypothalamus are all involved during the sexual stimulation of orgasm. Biologically and chemically speaking, sexual activity can be very reinforcing, and for the person who has crossed the line into sex addiction, recovery is possible but understandably difficult. Treatment focuses on establishing behavioral control and helping the sex addict to develop a healthy perspective of sexuality through education and psychotherapy. Sex Addicts Anonymous is a twelve-step group specifically designed to address this addiction and offers group support. Medications such as Prozac, Anafranil, and others used to treat obsessive-compulsive symptoms may be helpful in managing the obsessive nature of this disorder.

Essential

Although sex addicts may become involved in illegal sexual activities, it is important to recognize that this is not inevitable. A sex addict is not doomed to become a sexual offender. Sex addiction is highly associated with risk-taking and then blaming others for the resulting problems.

Relationships from a Distance: Cybersex

Internet sex, otherwise known as cybersex, is any sexual activity conducted via the Internet. Is cybersex automatically addictive? It can be. Approximately 8 to 10 percent of individuals who engage in cybersex become addicted.

Cybersex includes viewing pornography, reading and writing sexually explicit material, e-mailing to set up meetings with the intent of a sexual encounter, advertising to meet sexual partners, participating in sex-themed chat rooms, and engaging in interactive online affairs. Electronic cameras are frequently attached to the computer so that real-time viewing of another engaged in sexual activity is possible. Masturbation frequently accompanies Internet sexual viewing.

It has been estimated that as much as 60 percent of visits to the Internet have a sexual component. Many of the sexual acts engaged in online would be illegal if carried out in real life.

How can one determine if cybersex has become an addiction? Check out these signs:

- A cybersex addict spends excessive amounts of time online involved in sexual behaviors.
- As with other addictions, there will have been failed attempts to stop the behavior.
- An addict will become very frustrated or angry when asked to give up his online sexual involvements.
- Use of the Internet for sexual purposes interferes with an addict's work, school, or family time.
- An addict will become secretive and lie about his online sexual activity.
- Involvement in online affairs negatively affects a real-life relationship or marriage.
- An addict will increasingly limit his sexual activity to the Internet, avoiding real-life relationships altogether.

 Alert

Unsupervised children and adolescents may gain access to Internet pornography and cybersex that can be damaging to their mental, emotional, and sexual health. Additionally, the Internet has become a hunting ground for sexual predators who may lie and deceive their way into gaining access to unsuspecting, innocent children and adolescents. Monitor and protect your children!

All of the triggers and reinforcements that love and sex addicts experience in real life can be experienced by cybersex addicts as well. However, cybersex attracts people who would never consider aberrant or harmful sexual activity without the anonymity of the Internet. Many delude themselves into thinking that they avoid many of the risks of real-life sex, such as the physical risks of sexually transmitted diseases or assault. But other risks are quite present. A person may lose her job if caught engaging in cybersex on work time. Marriages and real-life relationships may be damaged when partners discover the cybersex and feel betrayed. If a cybersex addict is engaging in online sexual behaviors with minors, arrest and imprisonment are real-life possibilities. Psychotherapy and support groups can help. Recovery is always possible, but it takes the courage to admit to the problem and commitment to getting help.

Chat Room Addiction

A chat room is a way of conferencing with another person or a group of people online. This is accomplished with instant-messaging or text-messaging technology. Video cameras attached to the computer can also be used in chat room communications. Visual chat rooms may use added graphics with 2D or 3D virtual reality technology.

Chat rooms are prime targets for the initiation of cybersex. Can chat rooms be addictive? Yes, in the same way that other behaviors can become addictive. What are some of the warning signs? Here are a few:

- A chat room addict will find herself giving more personal details in chat rooms than she intended.
- Even when not in a chat room, a person will fantasize about chat room interactions.
- A person's sleep and eating behaviors will be disrupted because of time spent in the chat room.
- Real-life relationships suffer because of inordinate amounts of time spent in chat rooms.
- A chat room addict will become defensive and irritable when confronted about the time she spends on the computer.

Chat rooms, like cybersex, provide the illusion of safety and anonymity. Again, one must be careful of online predators and the personal risks of chat room addiction, such as job loss, lost relationships, and damage to one's personal health.

The Danger of Relational Addictions

There are many dangers involved in the relational addictions, some of them obvious and some not. Some of the obvious dangers from relational addictions include the risks to physical health, the potential loss of jobs, and even the risk of legal consequences and imprisonment.

Essential

Regardless of whether relationship addictions involve real people or virtual people, genuine emotions may develop. Too often, words said online are taken at face value when in fact, approximately 50 percent of Internet users have admitted to lying online. Love addicts tend to feel their emotions intensely, and thus hurt intensely when relationships are broken.

A less obvious danger of Internet relationship addictions is missed opportunities to form genuine, real-life relationships. Regardless of whether a relationship is casual or serious in nature, the development of healthy interactions requires a person's presence and intentional effort. Relationship addictions can be a way of escaping real-life relational problems. Personal growth in many areas of one's life (physical, emotional, spiritual, social, intellectual, and occupational) can be sidetracked with relationship addictions.

Talking to a Loved One about His or Her Problem

Denial, justification, and rationalization are just as prevalent in relationship addictions as in other addictions. Therefore, when approaching a friend or loved one about her problem, be prepared. Again, remember that this is not personal. It is evidence of the power and control that the addiction has over the addict. An individual with a relationship addiction may feel intense guilt and shame over her problem. Be gentle and compassionate with this, and remind the person of her strengths. Capitalizing on her strengths is what will help the relationship addict conquer her addiction. At the same time, direct honesty and firmness will be required to break through the barriers of denial.

Alert

> Human beings were made to be social and sexual. Even though relationship addictions do not provide healthy or satisfactory interactions with others, a relationship addict will fear the loss of what he has. Therefore, when encouraging a relationship addict to begin recovery, reassure him that he will not be abandoned or alone in his recovery.

Support groups can be particularly effective in helping an individual with relationship addictions. If necessary, offer to go with your friend or loved one. Helping with babysitting or transportation is another means of providing support. First and foremost, the relationship addict needs a friend and/or family member who will demonstrate and share healthy personal connections.

Seeking Help

If you have a relationship addiction or you care for someone who has, the first step in getting help is admitting the problem. This may very well be the most difficult aspect of recovery, as a relationship addiction may closely mimic what we accept as healthy. An evaluation by a mental health professional may help to assess the problem and determine a course of treatment. A psychiatric evaluation may provide the medical treatment that a co-occurring mental illness will require. Support groups can provide the reassurance that one is not "crazy" or "unlovable." The addicted person will see that she is not alone in dealing with these problems. Healthy relationships are not just good, they are necessary. And they take practice. The more exposure an addicted person can get to healthy relational models with opportunities to practice, the faster and more thoroughly she can enjoy recovery.

CHAPTER 13

Pornography Addiction

PORNOGRAPHY ADDICTION IS a form of sex addiction. However, it is so overwhelmingly prevalent and controversial in today's society that it deserves more in-depth treatment. Many say that pornography is an outgrowth of a person's natural desire to enjoy the human body and sex. Others declare that pornography is damaging to individuals involved and tears families apart. Regardless of where one stands on this debate, most people would agree that a pornography addiction can consume one's life.

Don't All Men Like to Look?

The popular notion of male sexuality is that men are more attracted to visual stimuli than women. This is being confirmed with modern scientific research. Functional magnetic resonance imaging (fMRI) has been used to demonstrate that the amygdala and hypothalamus are both more strongly activated in men than women when the same sexually arousing material is viewed by both sexes. You may recall that the amygdala is one of the primary brain areas making up the hedonic highway or pleasure pathway.

It has been discovered that when the amygdala is stimulated, there is an associated anticipation of positive emotions. In this case, there is an anticipation of the positive emotions, or pleasures, connected with sexual behavior. So when a man visually notices a woman he finds attractive, the parts of his brain involved in visual processing and arousal are activated. Once sexual climax has been reached, activity in the amygdala begins to decrease. There is some evidence that a larger amygdala may produce a more intense sex drive. Although a woman can also be sexually aroused by visual images, it is not typically to the same extent as with a man. A woman who is sexually aroused will typically show more activity in the areas of the brain associated with emotions. Women also seem to be more sexually aroused by smell or certain body odors than men.

Alert

> The novelty and uncertainty produced by pornographic images can become addicting. However, as the "newness" wears off and the pornographic images become common-place, the chemical stimulation of the pleasure circuits in the brain diminishes. Tolerance has developed and to achieve the same "high," exposure to even more novel images must occur. Thus, pornography addiction becomes a progressive disorder.

In addition to arousal, pornography has been shown to elicit fear, shame, anger, and lust in a significant number of people. Because of the nature of the stimulus, pornography, these other emotions may be mistakenly labeled as sexual arousal. Now combine this with memory. Visual images are more likely to be remembered than stimuli triggered by other senses. Additionally, the more novel and bizarre the visual image, the greater likelihood of its being stored in memory and recalled with vividness. The combination of fear, anxiety, and arousal produced by pornography often leads to confusion and the recall of visual images that can be interpreted as disturbing. This is dangerous in the minds of children with immature brains. The disturbing visual images of pornography, typically perceived with fear and anxiety, imprinted on a child's immature brain can lead to serious emotional and developmental damage.

In addition to the biological component of pornography, it is also asserted that men, primarily, are socialized in America to notice others sexually. Boys who find erotic magazines and view them are often seen as engaging in a normal rite of passage. Such activities are often met with snickers instead of instruction on developmentally healthy sexual behavior.

 Fact

> According to the National Center for Missing and Exploited Children, approximately 20 percent of all Internet pornography involves the use of children. In 2005, child pornography reportedly produced $3 billion of revenue.

Sex is used to sell products, and Americans have become conditioned to associate sexual images with many advertising campaigns. With sexual images so prevalent in society, it is no wonder that a person's amygdala can become aroused beyond what might be considered healthy.

 Question

> **What is the amygdala?**
> The amygdala, also known as the amygdaloid nucleus, is a small almond-shaped structure located in the temporal lobe of the brain. It is part of the brain's olfactory and limbic systems and is closely connected to the hypothalamus and hippocampus. The amygdala is involved in one's sense of smell, motivations, and emotional behaviors.

Entertainment or Addiction?

At the heart of the debate surrounding pornography is the question of whether pornography is simply entertainment enjoyed by consenting adults, or whether it is a truly harmful activity that may even lead to addiction. First of all, one must ask if pornography meets the criteria of an addiction.

Pornography, as with other addictions, follows a predictable behavioral cycle. A person becomes preoccupied with pornography and, as use increases, so does tolerance. A pornography addict will feel compelled to engage in this activity and may feel unable to control or stop the behavior. If a pleasure response is achieved, the addict will feel temporary relief. An addict who is unable to find pleasure or relief will experience frustration. When pornography is stopped, withdrawal symptoms will likely be experienced—irritability, anxiety, frustration, and so forth.

Essential

Healthy sexuality is an exciting, stimulating part of committed adult relationships. Sex, food, and spending can all become addictive and, because of their unavoidable presence in one's life, abstinence isn't always a solution. Changing one's thinking and behavioral processes from addictive back to controllable and healthy is difficult, but, often with help, can be accomplished.

Again, the brain is also involved as the addict's amygdala and the rest of the pleasure circuit stimulate arousal and the expectation of a pleasurable experience. The behavioral and physical reinforcements promote the continuation of the addictive cycle. How do you know if you are experiencing the symptoms of pornography addiction? Here are some questions to consider:

- Do sexual thoughts and/or behaviors monopolize your life to the exclusion of relationships and day-to-day responsibilities?
- Is it a struggle to control or stop your thinking about or viewing pornography?
- Have you lost your job or are you in danger of losing your job because of involvement with pornography?

- Do you spend more money on pornography than you can afford?
- Is it difficult to watch television or look at a magazine without flipping through the channels or pages looking for stimulating sexual material?
- Do you use pornography to escape, deny, or numb emotional problems?
- Do you feel the need to keep your pornography use secret or hidden?
- When confronted about pornography use, do you become angry, irritable, or offended?
- Has your pornography use continued despite negative consequences?
- After many attempts to stop pornography use, do you feel it is hopeless that you'll ever gain control of the problem?

If you have answered yes to many of these questions, then you have crossed the line from pornography as possibly entertaining to pornography as addictive. You will need help and extensive support to overcome the problem.

Unwilling Participants

Back to the debate over whether pornography can be entertainment between consenting adults. While that may be the case in a minority of instances, it is a fact that many who become involved in pornography are unwilling. A significant number of individuals associated with pornography have had a history of abuse, primarily sexual abuse. Nine out of ten children aged eight to sixteen have viewed pornography on the Internet. Many of these children inadvertently type in a trigger word that brings up pornographic material that they never intended to view. It has been estimated that one in seven children who use the Internet have received unwanted sexual solicitations while online. Runaways and victims of sexual abuse may become involved in pornography through no desire of their own. Either they see this as a means of financial survival or the victimized thinking from abuse makes them easy targets. These are not instances of consent.

Also, remember that visual stimuli have the most powerful effect on the brain. Visual stimuli can overwhelm the parts of the brain that control thinking and logic. Thus, the visual images of pornography may incapacitate the brain's ability to think and make informed consent regarding pornography use. It can also be argued that once pornography becomes an addiction, consent is eliminated with the loss of control associated with addiction.

What's the Problem with Admiring the Opposite Sex?

There is nothing wrong with admiring the opposite sex when it is age appropriate and causes no emotional, physical, mental, spiritual, or social harm to either person. It is unclear whether pornography can fit that criteria.

Both men and women enjoy the stimulating feelings of romantic attraction. In addition to the amygdala and hypothalamus already mentioned, the vagus nerves, the reticular formation, basal ganglia, anterior insular cortex, and cerebellum are all parts of the brain activated with sexual stimulation. And it has been said that frequent sexual orgasms can have beneficial effects such as lowering risk for heart attacks, release of endorphins, reduction in depressive symptoms, a calming effect, boost to the immune system, increased longevity, and a release of oxytocin and dehydroepiandrosterone (DHEA), which may inhibit the development of breast cancer. Along with these physical benefits of sexuality comes the emotional connectedness enjoyed by couples in a relationship. Pornography addiction overshadows these benefits by taking control of one's life, eliminating the relational component, and introducing unpleasant emotions such as shame and guilt.

The Effects of Pornography on Relationships

Individuals struggling with a pornography addiction often have difficulty developing and maintaining healthy, positive relationships. In some cases, there may be a fear or inability to bond and commit to a real-life relationship. Physical and emotional intimacy may feel very frightening to the pornography addict. If an individual has grown up in a family where commitments were not honored and trust was not developed, she may not believe that these things are possible for her as an adult, either. Pornography presents a person with relationship illusions, seemingly without the risk of disappointment, failure, or abandonment.

 Fact

> Pornography has been identified as a significant problem in American families. One 2003 survey suggested that as many as 47 percent of the families questioned identified pornography as a problem in their homes. Pornography addiction is leading more and more couples into therapy for help and is also becoming a significant factor in many divorces.

For many who discover that their partner has a pornography addiction, feelings of shock, confusion, and betrayal are typical reactions. These feelings may be just as deep and real as if the object of the partner's affections were a real-life person and an actual affair had occurred. Pornography addiction is often considered an affair of the mind by the person's partner, so the implications of these feelings are often quite similar to those of an actual affair. In a marriage or committed relationship, trust may be severely damaged and the sexual relationship may become difficult or impossible to sustain. Partners of the pornography addict frequently claim that the secretiveness, the lying, and the betrayal are worse to handle than the pornography itself. The pornography addict, who may have distanced himself emotionally from his real-life relationships, frequently finds this reaction to his addiction difficult to understand. This creates further conflict in the relationship. For the partner of the addict, it may be difficult to comprehend that pornography addiction is not about sexual or relational intimacy. Pornography addiction, as with other addictions, is often about escaping emotional problems and achieving a biochemical "high."

Essential

Even though pornography may not involve real-life sexual partners, real-life feelings are strong and powerful. Anger, jealousy, fear, depression, anxiety, and hurt may have a significant effect on the partner of the pornography addict. The partner of a pornography addict may need professional treatment to deal with these emotions, just as the addict will likely need professional treatment for recovery.

An individual who is addicted to pornography very likely has a public image of normalcy and respectability. The pornography addict's partner may fear how exposure of the pornography addiction could affect the family in the community. If the addict is engaging in pornography in the workplace, the possibility of job loss and the economic impact that would have on the family may be quite real. Both individual and couples psychotherapy will likely be required to work through the complexities that this addiction creates.

Legal Implications

The legal implications surrounding pornography can be complex. For example, the question may arise as to whether pornography and prostitution are connected. According to the U.S. Supreme Court, pornographic actors are protected by the First Amendment as long as obscenity is not involved. Even though the pornographic actors may themselves be involved in actual sex, the consumer of pornography is not and therefore is also legally protected. The whole legal picture changes when children are involved. Child pornography is illegal in every state. In 2001, laws were established prohibiting child pornography on the Internet.

Alert

> As of 2003, it was estimated that 20,000 images of child pornography were posted on the Internet every week. Although child pornography is illegal in every state, some states go even further to try to protect children. South Carolina, for instance, requires computer technicians to report any child pornography they encounter in their work to law enforcement officials.

In July of 2006, the Organization for Security and Cooperation in Europe (OSCE) adopted a United States–sponsored resolution condemning the sexual exploitation of children. This resolution, "Combating Trafficking and the Exploitation of Children in Pornography," requires the participating members to ensure criminal prosecution for the production or dissemination of child pornography. In 2003, the U.S. Immigration and Customs Enforcement developed an initiative in cooperation with other OSCE member states to investigate and prosecute pedophiles, Internet predators, human traffickers, international sex tourists, and other predatory criminals. With the advent of the world wide web, it has become evident that problems with pornography addiction and the associated criminal element is an international issue.

Treatment for the Addict

Treatment for a pornography addict may very well require professional guidance and, certainly, a strong system of support. In reality, there is nowhere in our society that a pornography addict can go and not encounter sexual triggers. As with food addiction, abstinence is generally not an option. Therefore, a pornography addict will need to learn to control the addictive, compulsive impulses and to retrain his thinking about sexuality. Common examples of dysfunctional beliefs that a pornography addict may buy into include:

- I am unlovable the way I am.
- It is not possible to have my needs met with another person.
- Sex is the most important need in my life.
- The sexual desires I have are bad and unforgivable. Therefore, I must satisfy them in secret.

Cognitive-behavioral psychotherapy can be helpful in changing these self-destructive thought patterns.

 Question

What are antiandrogens?
Antiandrogens are medications that inhibit the biological effects of androgens. Androgens are sex hormones. Antiandrogens may reduce sexual urges, erections, and fantasies. Typically, these medications are used in more extreme cases when the compulsive sexual behavior may be harmful to others. A pedophile who lures children into pornography might be a candidate for this type of treatment.

If the Internet has been a vehicle for pornography, there are many blocking and filtering programs that can be purchased for installation on one's computer. These programs are helpful for the addict who wants to resist temptation and also for protecting kids from viewing pornographic material. Twelve-step support groups such as Sex Addicts Anonymous (SAA), Sex and Love Addicts Anonymous (S.L.A.A.), and Sexaholics Anonymous (SA), have also been helpful. Each addict will need to identify her particular triggers and devise strategies to manage her responses or to avoid the triggers. As with other addictions, pharmacological treatment for obsessive thinking and/or for co-occurring mental health problems may be beneficial. Medications that have been used to treat compulsive sexual behavior include selective serotonin reuptake inhibitors (SSRIs) such as fluoxetine (Prozac), paroxetine (Paxil), sertraline (Zoloft), and others. In addition to treating the compulsivity, the medications themselves often cause sexual side effects such as lowered libido. Mood stabilizers such as lithium, antianxiety medications, and naltrexone have also been used.

Support for Partners of Pornography Addicts

The spouses and committed partners of pornography addicts also will likely require treatment themselves to recover from the fallout. If trust has been broken with the addict, it may be helpful to engage in individual or group therapy for emotional healing prior to working on rebuilding the relationship. Since it is so easy to take this addiction personally, it is important for the partner of the addict to educate himself regarding pornography addiction. There may be a tendency for the partner of the addict to feel he was somehow inadequate to meet the addict's sexual needs and that's why the addict turned to pornography. This isn't true. As previously discussed, pornography addiction is related to biochemistry and problems within the addict herself. Healthy self-care, the support of friends and family, as well as psychotherapy will help the partner cope and maintain his own healthy self-image. Recovery for the pornography addict, the partner, and the relationship is possible!

CHAPTER 14

Technology and Addiction

TECHNOLOGY IS THE application of science and the scientific method to achieve a commercial goal. Inventions like the telegraph, telephone, and electric light bulb began to excite imaginations about what might be accomplished through the use of science. Technological advances have taken the human population way beyond expectations. Fantasies and dreams have become reality—man has walked on the moon and information from around the world is at one's fingertips through computers the size of credit cards. Addictions associated with technology have also become a reality.

The New Complication in Addictions

Technology itself is the latest addiction. The complication created by technology addiction is the difficulty one has in sorting out what is necessary, what is utilitarian, what is convenience, what is entertainment, and when the line is crossed into addiction. Being technologically savvy can affect your ability to communicate, to get a job, to keep a job, to be socially acceptable, and to complete your education. An additional complication created by technology is the development of a whole new language and vocabulary. Anyone who can't speak "technologese" can quickly feel isolated in society.

So how does someone know if he's crossed the line from being technologically on top of things to addiction? Here are some clues:

- He becomes incapable of managing his time on the computer, the BlackBerry, the iPod, and so forth.
- He has a feeling of euphoria while using his technological device of choice.
- He begins lying to family, friends, or his employer about the time spent on technological devices.
- He abandons real-life hobbies, social interactions, and productive pursuits in order to spend more time with his technological addictions.
- He develops health issues relating to technology addiction: carpal tunnel syndrome, eyestrain, dry eyes, migraines, poor personal hygiene, sleep disorders, weight gain, and backaches.
- He becomes irritable, angry, or upset if interrupted while involved with his technological devices.
- He feels guilt and shame over spending more time with technology than his family and friends.
- He decides to cut down on technology use, tries, but repeatedly fails.
- He will begin to crave more and more time with his technology "substance" and become frustrated if his time is denied.

Many of these signs and symptoms of technology addiction are familiar variations on the signs of other addictions. Again, the common theme is loss of control and negative consequences in one's life as a result of the addiction.

The Dangers of Technology Addiction

Technology addiction can lead to other dangerous consequences. The speed with which technology moves makes everything available within seconds or less. This promotes a desire for instant gratification. Everything seems to be marked "urgent" and the expectation is that the request will be immediately granted. Sleep disorders can develop as a person stays up all hours of the night to play video games, answer e-mails, instant-message with friends, or download music. Weight gain and other complications of a sedentary lifestyle such as cardiovascular disease may result. Learning and practicing social skills with live people may suffer, especially in the case of children and teens who spend an inordinate amount of time in front of the television or computer. Technology addictions may also give someone a false sense of relational security as he communicates with individuals around the world whom he will never meet in person.

Dependency is created, and when the technological substance of choice is removed or denied, withdrawal symptoms ensue. Frustration, anxiety, anger, and fear are common symptoms of withdrawal from technology.

Essential

Technology in the twenty-first century is unavoidable. In fact, most jobs and careers require technological knowledge on some level to function. However, the novelty of technological devices can stimulate an addictive response in susceptible individuals. It can be difficult for an addict to function appropriately with technology use, keeping it within the bounds of what's required.

It's the Latest!

Some individuals may become as obsessed with obtaining the latest in technology as with using it. It becomes a status symbol, and long lines may form with people waiting for hours in inclement weather just to be the first through the door as sales of the newest device begin. Of course, advertising around the latest in technology is huge and geared to trigger even the mildest inclination toward addiction into a full-scale purchasing frenzy. For a true technology addict, this spells danger. It is quite easy to lose control of good judgment, and debt can mount to compound the problem of addiction. The latest in technology always means top-dollar prices.

Video Game Addiction

Video games encompass a wide variety of interests. Cartoon-like games for children, card games such as solitaire, puzzle games, and interactive role-playing games make video games a temptation for all ages.

 Fact

Solitaire addiction was cited as a problem costing millions of dollars in state government in 2005. North Carolina State Senator Austin Allran proposed antisolitaire legislation claiming that state government employees were spending too much time playing solitaire and neglecting their work. His request was that all games be erased from computers used by the state.

Some games require a one-time purchase, some can be accessed for free, and others require a monthly fee to play. Apart from games on the Internet, video game systems such as Nintendo, Xbox, and now Wii can be purchased to use in conjunction with a television screen. There is no question that playing games can be fun and entertaining, a release from the stresses of life. When does playing video games become a problem? Asking these questions may help evaluate whether playing video games is problematic:

- How many hours a day do you spend gaming? Are necessary daily functions falling by the wayside because of excessive time spent gaming?
- Do thoughts about the video game dominate your mind when involved in other activities such as work or school?
- Do you pretend to go to bed, then get up to play a video game after others are asleep?
- Are you skipping school or work to play video games?
- Does gaming "language" start to become part of your real-life conversations?

- Do you have an over-identification with one's gaming character? Do you consistently try to think and behave as you believe the gaming character would?
- Do you lose whole nights of sleep because of gaming?
- Do you have more of a connection with online gaming friends than real-life relationships?
- Have you made multiple attempts to cut back or stop playing video games without success? Do you feel guilty about the failures to control time spent gaming?

If the answer to several of these questions is yes, you may begin to question whether a serious problem is developing. Addiction to gaming is real and can take over a person's life. Is video game addiction just a behavioral problem or a failure to manage one's priorities, or are there physiological components as well? For many, this is the criteria for whether a substance or behavior is truly an addiction.

☐⌙ Essential

Other mental disorders such as obsessive-compulsive disorder, depressive disorders, and anxiety disorders may coexist with technology addictions. Attention deficit hyperactivity disorder (ADHD) is one such disorder that puts a potential addict at risk. Video games in particular provide immediate gratification and tremendous stimulation to one's brain. A person with ADHD finds this stimulation and reinforcement hard to resist.

Research is demonstrating that, once again, brain chemistry is involved. Excessive game playing has been shown to increase the release of dopamine in the brain just as with other addictive substances and behaviors. Once this occurs, there is the same resulting feelings of euphoria. Memory becomes involved and the brain remembers the pleasure experienced while playing games, reinforcing the desire to play again and again.

Hazards of Video Games

Video games have an additional effect on the brain that other addictions do not. Brain waves have been shown to be negatively affected by video games, specifically alpha and beta waves. Alpha waves are involved in imagery and relaxation or rest. Beta waves indicate increased activity in the prefrontal lobe of the brain, which is the center of emotion and creativity. Alpha waves can be artificially produced through exposure to radiant light emanating from computer monitors or televisions. This can begin to happen within thirty seconds of focusing on the screen. Typically, alpha waves are present when one's eyes are closed, such as when a person is daydreaming. A person's brain does not function as intended when alpha waves occur during wakefulness with eyes opened. This condition tends to put a person in an unfocused, receptive state similar to that induced through hypnosis.

 Alert

Parents need to monitor what children see on video games. The Entertainment Software Rating Board (ESRB) provides video game ratings to give consumers information about the content of the game and recommendations on age-appropriateness. Rating categories include Early Childhood (EC), Everyone (E), Teen (T), Mature (M), Adults Only (AO), and Rating Pending. Every rating category except EC may contain violent material.

Beta waves are present when the mind is fully engaged in active mental processes. Individuals who play few to no video games generally have much stronger beta waves than alpha waves. However, excessive gamers who spend several hours per day playing video games, may display little to no beta wave activity. The startling fact is that this absence of beta wave activity persists even when the person has stopped playing. It has been noted that when this occurs, a person exhibits difficulty concentrating, irritability, and problems socializing with real-life people.

Another hazard with video games relates to one's exposure to violence. Many video games, particularly those involving role-playing, contain violent content. For a video game addict who experiences excessive exposure to violence, the danger of becoming desensitized to real-life violence is of genuine concern. Research has demonstrated that someone who has played a violent video game for even twenty minutes will have significantly reduced physiological responses to real-life violence. Typically, a person's heart rate will increase and her skin's responses will increase when exposed to violence.

It appears that playing violent video games causes a person to become physiologically numb with lowered heart rate and skin responses. It has also been demonstrated that a person playing violent video games has less activity in the prefrontal area of the brain, which is involved in concentration, self-control, and inhibition. Instead, the amygdala is stimulated leading to increased emotional arousal. With the numbers of individuals playing video games in our society, this information is of great concern socially.

Addiction to Cell Phones and Other Technological Devices

Cell phones have become standard apparatus in twenty-first-century existence. It has been estimated that American cell phone subscribers have increased from 38 million to 219 million since 1996. Cell phones are seen as a requirement by many in our world of technological communication. Can cell phone usage become addictive? More and more people believe it can. Dependence has developed on cell phones such that many individuals describe feeling insecure, anxious, and fearful if required to turn the cell phone off. What are signs that cell phone use is problematic? Here are a few:

- Cell phone bills that cause financial hardships
- Encountering negative consequences at school and work because of cell phone use

- Feeling a constant need to be on the cell phone
- Relationship problems due to excessive time on the cell phone
- Using a cell phone at times when it's dangerous to do so, such as in heavy traffic
- Cell phone usage continues to escalate
- Irritation and frustration when others request getting off the cell phone
- Obsessive behavior related to cell phone usage

Talking about the latest in technology, cell phones are now capable of many more functions than conversation. In reality, they have become minicomputers with which a person can access e-mail, plan her day, play games, and watch a movie.

 Fact

Cell phone usage while driving is considered dangerous by many—so much so that state legislatures are taking action. Five states, the District of Columbia, and the Virgin Islands prohibit hand-held cell phone usage while driving. Seventeen states and the District of Columbia ban cell phone use by novice drivers. Many states ban cell phone use in specific circumstances.

Believe it or not, cell phones also affect one's brain. Cell phones send off electromagnetic fields that excite the brain. The cortical area of the brain, which is responsible for movement and language, is stimulated when exposed to cell phone usage. Research into the physiological effects of cell phones is still in the infancy stage, and at this point it is unknown whether the effects are enough to cause damage.

The list of technological devices available for work, communication, and/or entertainment is almost endless. MP3 players are devices that compress music, meaning they reduce the amount of computerized space required to store a song. While a compact disc may have twelve to sixteen songs per disc, an MP3 player can store hundreds of songs. An iPod is a portable media player that allows one to store photos, play videos, games, music, and manage calendars, among other things. A BlackBerry device can be used to e-mail, phone, map, organize, game, and access the Internet. The Wii is a new interactive gaming system that attaches to a television set. Individuals can use it to play games online or live, alone or with others.

Essential

The American Psychiatric Association and the American Medical Association are considering whether video game addiction is a legitimate diagnosis. A new *Diagnostic and Statistical Manual of Mental Disorders* is scheduled for release in 2012. There is no agreement concerning the diagnosis at this time. However, the compulsive nature of gaming is unquestionable in certain individuals and should be closely monitored.

This is just a sampling of the technological devices available. In terms of addiction, they all have the potential of taking control of a person's life.

Internet Addiction

It has been estimated that the average Internet user spends about three and a half hours online each day. Five to ten percent of online users are said to be addicted to the Internet. So what is Internet addiction? Internet addiction has been described as an impulse-control disorder that is similar in nature to gambling addiction. Internet addiction includes gaming, pornography, shopping, chatting, and so on. Although many question whether Internet addiction is a true addiction or simply problematic behavior, for some users it can meet certain addiction criteria: needing more and more to maintain satisfaction, and experiencing irritability and discomfort when stopped. There can definitely be an obsessive and compulsive use of the Internet. As with other addictions, excessive Internet use can stimulate the release of dopamine and the pleasure derived from that encourages further use.

Alert

Single people and young adults are cited as most likely to be using the Internet. Social networking, dating using websites, updating personal web pages, e-mailing, and instant messaging, among other things, are common activities. While this sounds harmless enough, it translates into consistently and significantly less time spent with family and friends, lost time studying for school, and lost time on the job.

The following signs suggest that an Internet user may be in danger of becoming addicted:

- She becomes preoccupied with and obsessed about using the Internet.
- She experiences feelings of restlessness, moodiness, anxiety, depression, or irritability when she attempts to cut down on Internet use or is questioned about her use by others.
- Internet use is putting her job or schoolwork in jeopardy.
- She becomes increasingly isolated from real-life relationships.
- Physical symptoms from excessive Internet use appear, such as sleep disorders, eating disorders, headaches, backaches, carpal tunnel syndrome, and eye disorders.
- She lies about her Internet use, which creates problems with family members and friends.
- She uses the Internet to escape uncomfortable emotions or problems.

- She has attempted multiple times to cut down usage without success.
- She experiences feelings of guilt related to her excessive Internet use.

A person at risk for Internet addiction is one who may have problems developing satisfying relationships with others. She may feel insecure or inadequate to handle life in the real world. The Internet can offer a virtual or make-believe community in which an addict can deny and repress her real-life problems.

 Question

What is virtual reality?
Virtual reality can best be described as an illusion of the real world simulated or created by a computer system. This can occur in one's imagination, or special gear can be used to heighten the experience. Special glasses and headphones create a greater sensation of sight and sound. Gloves with electronic sensors can also be used to touch or move virtual objects.

Illusions can be very powerful, especially when mixed with use that may be legitimate. The Internet is a requirement for many facets of work and life in our current age. For an addict, however, required Internet use blends into an uncontrollable and unmanageable life problem.

The Lure of Anonymity

Anonymity is both attractive and a problem for the technology addict. For someone with social skills deficits, self-image problems, and/or low self-esteem, anonymity provided by technology seems to be a blessing. Online friends, for example, never need to know what one looks like, sounds like, or acts like. All identifying information can be transformed so that a person can be anyone she wants. This can allow the technology addict to avoid working on personal growth through interaction and practice with real people. Anonymity is not just dangerous because a person can avoid facing painful emotions and situations, it can also be a cover for predators. It is well known that sexual predators, in particular, use the anonymity of technology to attract their victims and avoid detection. Financial scams are also frequently perpetrated through the anonymity of technology.

Fact

Internet scams are varied, convincing, and dangerous in their pursuit of stealing money and the identities of potential victims. Killer or hitman e-mails are blackmail schemes in which the sender poses as an assassin demanding money for safety. Many Internet scams were developed to take advantage of donors wanting to help Hurricanes Katrina and Rita victims. Take time to investigate any suspicious Internet message.

Credit card fraud, blackmail schemes, lottery winner scams, and even relief fund fraud abound in the world of virtual crime. Addicts who are already excessively pulled into the use of technology are prime targets, as are children and adults who are not as fluent in the use and language of technology.

Talking to a Loved One about His or Her Problem

Technological interests can become so mesmerizing that getting one's attention may be the initial challenge in talking with a friend or loved one about this problem. Don't be put off by a person's irritability at being pulled away from her addiction. The irritability and frustration over being interrupted is part of the disorder and exactly why a discussion is necessary.

Gently say to the addict that you believe a problem exists and it's important to talk. Reinforce this with reassurance that criticism or judgment is not the object of the conversation, but rather your concern over his deteriorating condition. The addict's emotional, psychological, spiritual, social, and physical health are the focus of the confrontation. Remember that symptoms of withdrawal are real and uncomfortable. Offer to help the person through this time by making yourself available to engage in other fun and meaningful activities. Re-establishing connections with real-life people and developing satisfying relationships will be the best medicine in helping the addict overcome this problem. If all else fails, a formal intervention process with friends and family involved may be necessary to help the addict begin to realize how much the addiction is affecting her life and the lives of those who care about her. Stating the facts of the effects of the addiction, not personal attacks, is the goal of an intervention. Interventions need to end with offers of help, support, and encouragement.

Essential

Unmet emotional needs often lead a potential addict to pursue technology for the appearance of relational interaction. The most helpful intervention friends and family members can do is to engage in genuine and heartfelt experiences with the addict. If a mental health disorder with emotional problems is co-occurring with the technology addiction, encourage the addict to seek professional treatment.

Seeking Help

Thinking of technology as a possible addiction is a new approach in the field of addiction treatment. Gambling, pornography, and spending have been researched and have gained credibility as potentially addictive behaviors.

Many times when someone wonders if she has a technology addiction, there is a fear of not being taken seriously or even being made the butt of a joke. This could be the first hurdle to jump over in seeking help. As with other addictions, support groups have developed around technology addictions. A few of these groups include Internet Addicts Anonymous, Gaming Addiction, and Internet Addicts Recovery Club. Technology doesn't have to take over a person's life. Recovery is possible and a person can regain control.

Question

Are there treatment programs specifically for technology addictions?

Yes, specialized programs targeting technology addictions do exist, but at this time, they are few in number. To locate a program, ask a mental health professional for help. One thing to remember is that since technology addiction is not yet a recognized mental health disorder diagnosis, it is unlikely that insurance will pay for this type of treatment.

CHAPTER 15

Roadblocks to Treatment

RECOVERY FROM ADDICTIONS is very difficult to achieve solo. Addictions are complicated disorders involving every aspect of a person's life. They also have significant effects on anyone connected to the addict. It seems logical that anyone experiencing the devastating effects of an addiction would desire help through treatment and a return to healthy living. However, there are many reasons why someone might avoid treatment. Roadblocks to treatment must be faced and removed before beginning the path to recovery.

Dealing with Denial

Without a doubt, denial is the most significant roadblock to recovery. Denial is a defense mechanism, a reaction to protect oneself from the truth of addiction. Lying about one's addiction or refusing to discuss the subject may be the first indicators of denial. At this stage of denial, the addict may recognize that his substance use or behavior is a problem, but may not recognize the depth of its effects. As time goes on and problems mount related to his addiction, denial becomes a means of psychological survival. Although denial is typically an unconscious process, it is the most common method an addict uses to manage his fears.

There are many fears that may strike deeply into the heart of an addict. He may fear others finding out about his addiction; he may fear the legal and financial consequences of his behavior catching up to him; he may fear the loss of relationships over his addiction;

and most of all, he may fear withdrawal and life without the addiction. Denial says that if the problem is not acknowledged, it doesn't exist. The painful thoughts, the emotional conflicts, and the anxiety surrounding the addiction are simply someone else's problem. If others would stop bothering the addict, everything would be fine. Those who love and care for the addict recognize that this isn't true, but one must realize that she is highly invested in maintaining his state of denial. There is a great deal at stake in admitting the truth about addiction. Recall that addictions are commonly used to manage painful and difficult emotions and/or psychological problems. To give up denial, an addict has to find another way to deal with his problems. Denial of addiction may also be related to denial of other mental health problems. The layers of fear and anxiety in an addict's life may go deeper than one might think.

 Fact

> It has been estimated that over 4.5 million Americans meet criteria for needing drug and alcohol addiction treatment, but deny they have a problem. These statistics include people aged twelve and older. It is of great concern that teenagers make up a significant portion of those individuals in denial of their need for help.

There are specific indicators that a person is in denial about his addiction. Here are some common ones:

- Refusing to learn the facts about the effects of addiction
- Distorting information related to his addiction such as the amount or frequency of usage
- Minimizing the significance of his use of an addictive substance or compulsive behaviors
- Lying to friends and family members as well as himself about the extent and details of his addiction

- Selective memory related to his addiction, acknowledging only those details related to his addiction that would not raise alarm, such as going out with friends to a party and neglecting to include that alcohol and cocaine were the focus of the party
- "Euphoric recall" or remembering only the good times associated with the addiction
- Wishful thinking related to his addiction such as imagining he could engage in his addiction without negative consequences or that he could stop the addiction without problems any time he chooses
- Avoiding conversations related to his addiction

 Question

What are defense mechanisms?
Defense mechanisms are psychological processes, often unconscious, that allow a person to protect himself from real or perceived threats or stressful situations. Sigmund Freud first described the concept of defense mechanisms in 1894. His daughter, Anna Freud, continued work in this area in the 1930s. The most commonly recognized defense mechanisms are denial, repression, regression, sublimation, rationalization, projection, reaction formation, and displacement.

How should a person's denial be confronted? Carefully. Confronting an addict's denial too harshly or abruptly may only serve to drive him away from necessary treatment. Denial is not always a bad thing. It can be positive protection for a person who has experienced trauma or emotions too painful to acknowledge all at once. Denial is maladaptive when it persists and prevents a person from getting the help he needs. In addressing denial, one's fears need to be taken seriously and support provided. Allow the addict to freely talk about his fears in relation to his addiction. Irrational thoughts or beliefs the addict holds need to be identified and replaced with evidence of truth. For example, many addicts believe that the addiction is too powerful and that nothing will help. This is an irrational thought that can be replaced with truthful evidence of treatment options.

Essential

A person in denial about his addiction has often isolated himself from others, cutting himself off from objective information and feedback related to his addiction. A person's imagination can easily exaggerate information when in isolation. Exaggerated and distorted information can lead to further isolation. Being a friend and gently reminding the addict of reality can help.

Denial may also be covering up shame and guilt an addict feels. Attacking a person's denial by telling him he should be ashamed of how he's affected others and damaged himself is quite harmful. Confronting denial with attacks and "beating the addict down" creates further destruction that will need to be repaired before recovery can take place. Empathy and understanding, while at the same time telling the reality of what one sees, will reassure the addict that it is safe to face his denial. As an addict sorts through his fears and anxieties over addressing his addiction, he will need to experience acceptance and support. The person considering the need to confront the addict may need help in dealing with her own feelings of anger and resentment before she can be effective. This is understandable. Confronting denial around addictions is difficult for everyone concerned. Patience is most definitely a desirable quality in this situation.

Budgeting for Treatment

There is no question that addiction treatment can be expensive. However, there are ways to get help, and treatment is not nearly as expensive as the costs incurred by the addiction itself. Individually, the costs of unemployment, illness, and legal expenses related to addictions can be astronomical in comparison to the cost of treatment.

 Alert

The latest statistics indicate that 23.2 million Americans struggle with addictions. Shockingly, only about 10 percent are receiving the treatment they need. The stigma of having an addiction, the cost of treatment, and fear of losing one's job are reasons commonly cited for avoiding treatment. While understandable, these are all obstacles that must, and can, be overcome.

Nationally, the costs of addiction may exceed a half trillion dollars annually when one considers health care expenditures, lost productivity on the job, and the costs resulting from criminal activity. There are some encouraging trends when it comes to funding addiction treatments. Health care insurance is one major way that an individual can fund his addiction treatment. A person with health insurance benefits would be responsible for a co-pay determined by the insurance company.

In July 2007, the House Education and Labor Committee voted to approve a mental health and addiction parity bill called The Paul Wellstone Mental Health and Addiction Equity Act of 2007. This bill would require any group health plan having at least fifty members to cover addiction and mental health problems at the same level as medical illnesses. In September 2007, the U.S. Senate voted to approve the Mental Health Parity Act. The House passed a mental health parity bill in March 2008. Some differences need to be worked out yet and full congressional approval will be necessary before a national mental health parity law goes into effect. The primary differences in the two bills that will require clarification include specification of the range of diagnoses to be covered, the management of benefits by health plans, and how out-of-network benefits will be covered. Nevertheless, major progress has been made toward ending insurance discrimination against mental health and addiction treatment. It is expected that congressional action on this issue will occur late in 2008. On a state level, forty-three states and the District of Columbia have active laws requiring insurance companies to provide some kind of coverage for addiction treatment. However, many have encountered problems with insurance companies delaying or denying treatment and/or placing restrictions on addiction treatment benefits.

 Question

What is mental health parity?
Parity is making two things equal. In the case of mental health parity, this refers to creating equality in the health insurance industry between mental health coverage and medical health coverage. Currently, only about 1 to 2 percent of health care insurance dollars go toward paying for mental health care. Many mental health services are excluded or severely restricted by insurance companies.

If a person encounters problems getting her insurance company to pay for mental health care and/or addiction treatment, there are some things she can do:

- Know the details of her health care coverage.
- Check coverage as described in her employee benefit handbook. Her employer may be able to override or negotiate with the insurance company on her behalf.
- Contact the state insurance department, the health department, or even the Office of the Attorney General. These agencies have the power to enforce addiction treatment laws.
- Ask a local or state legislator to intervene on her behalf. These elected officials appropriate funding to state offices and have an interest in seeing laws enforced.

- Ask the administrators of health care facilities where treatment is being sought to help work with insurance companies.
- Document all interactions with her insurance company and keep copies of all correspondence.

If someone doesn't have health insurance, what are the costs of treatment and how does she pay? Although facilities certainly vary in what they charge, the average cost for a single course of outpatient addiction treatment, which lasts about six weeks, can start at around $1,500. Short-term residential treatment, typically lasting twenty days, may average approximately $4,000 per admission. Long-term residential treatment often lasts around ninety days. Costs can run much higher than this depending on the length of treatment and whether one attends a "no frills" program or one with all the luxuries.

All states have some funds for substance abuse prevention and addiction treatment for individuals who have no insurance or inadequate insurance. To find the agency in your state that manages these funds, go to *www.natlalliance.org*. Federal funds from the Temporary Assistance for Needy Families (TANF) program may be available for nonmedical drug and alcohol treatment. There is also the federal Welfare-to-Work program that may help fund individuals who are required to receive drug and alcohol abuse treatment in order to return to work. Again, the funds are only available for nonmedical treatment. Most treatment programs and individual providers also provide some pro bono services for those in need who have no other options.

Finally, some employers are now recognizing how helpful it is to their company to have healthy employees and are funding some treatment as a job benefit. Check it out with the human resource department. Don't be afraid to ask. Treatment is important and it is effective!

Finding the Right Treatment for You

No one treatment program is right for everyone. Each person has his own medical needs, social needs, legal and vocational issues, psychological needs, and spiritual needs. Financial concerns are also significant. It takes time to find the treatment program that is the best "fit." Be patient! Finding the right program will lead to the best opportunity for successful recovery.

The two basic types of treatment programs are residential/inpatient programs and outpatient programs. Within that framework, many variations are available, depending on the addict's particular needs and situation. Residential or inpatient hospital programs typically last for twenty-one to thirty days. These programs are appropriate for individuals who:

- Require medical supervision
- Are unresponsive to less restrictive forms of treatment
- Have inadequate support systems at home
- Have spiraled out of control with the addiction and need help to break the cycle

Alert

Remember that many individuals struggling with addiction have more than one addiction and/or other mental health problems. When choosing a treatment program, make certain that professionally trained staff are available to manage complex treatment issues if necessary. Programs targeting only one addiction, such as alcohol, will likely be unsuccessful and discourage the addict from seeking further treatment.

Outpatient programs typically last thirty to ninety days or even longer with support and maintenance. These programs are appropriate for individuals who:

- Have adequate support systems in place at home
- Can maintain a level of safety

- Are motivated for treatment
- Are medically stable

Several types of outpatient programs are available and a professional evaluation may be helpful to determine which will best meet the addict's needs. One such program is a partial hospitalization program or intensive day program. To be eligible for these programs, a person must be medically and psychiatrically stable with an adequate, supportive living situation. The programs last from two to eight hours per day, two to five days per week. Although they may take place in a hospital setting, the individual goes home at night and has the opportunity to practice coping skills in real-life situations.

 Question

What is a therapeutic community (TC)?
Therapeutic community is a specialized type of inpatient treatment. This highly structured residential treatment program is for an addict with a long history of severe addiction. The program often lasts six to twelve months and is designed to completely change the addict's lifestyle and equip him to successfully re-enter the job market and society.

Outpatient programs can be an excellent solution for someone who wants to maintain her employment and help meet family obligations. Some outpatient programs are primarily educational and supportive in nature. Group counseling is often a component of both inpatient and outpatient treatment. Some programs provide individual and family counseling as part of the package, or you may opt to find these services privately. Network therapy is a type of treatment that includes specified family members and friends who help the treatment team promote behavioral and attitudinal change on the part of the addict.

The most successful treatment programs are comprehensive, employ professionals who specialize in working with addictions and mental health disorders, and offer multiple levels of treatment to accommodate the changing needs of the addict. Comprehensive programs include vocational rehabilitation, parenting skills training, legal services, social skills training, educational services, spiritual support if desired, and aftercare programs.

Locating Qualified Professionals

Physicians, nurses, social workers, psychologists, and counselors may all have some knowledge of addictions. However, only a limited number among these groups will have specialized training, experience, and certification to treat addictions. How does one locate a qualified professional? There are many avenues to pursue. A person's health insurance company will have a list of qualified professionals for referral. Employee Assistance Programs (EAPs) will also be able to provide this information to employees. There are state chapters of the American Society of Addiction Medicine (ASAM) and the National Association of Alcoholism and Drug Abuse Counselors (NAADAC) that may be contacted for assistance. Some individuals prefer help for addictions through a spiritual leader. The American Association of Pastoral Counselors (AAPC) accredits pastoral counseling centers and can help locate a qualified person. The American Medical Association DoctorFinder program (*http://webapps.ama-assn.org/doctorfinder/home.html*) can be accessed to locate a physician specializing in addictions.

The National Register database (*www.nationalregister.com*) and/or the American Psychological Association (*www.apa.org*) are associations that can help locate psychologists who work with addictions. The American Nurses Association (*www.nursingworld.org*) and/or the International Nurses Society on Addictions (*www.intnsa.org*) are excellent resources for locating nurse practitioners who specialize in addiction treatment. Psychiatric hospitals, addiction treatment centers, and community mental health agencies will also have information about addiction treatment specialists in the community.

 Fact

An addictionologist is a physician who has received specialized training in the treatment of addictions. An addictionologist may be a doctor of medicine (M.D.) or a doctor of osteopathy (D.O.). This is a professional who is best qualified to treat the medical complications of addiction, prescribe medications for treatment, and recognize any complicating mental health disorders.

What if Treatment Threatens My Job?

The effects of addiction treatment on one's job are a widespread concern for many individuals. It is estimated that more than 25 percent of individuals struggling with addictions believe they would experience negative job consequences if they sought treatment. A person may fear losing a license necessary for his work, failing to get a promotion, losing authority with subordinates, or losing the respect of coworkers and supervisors. Shame and embarrassment are big factors that often prevent a person from approaching her employer or human resource director to request addiction treatment. In the current American economy, the fear of losing one's job and being unable to find another is a realistic concern.

It is up to employers to create an environment where getting help for addictions is not only acceptable, but also commendable. Employers can do this by informing new hires of addiction treatment benefits during orientation. This needs to be reviewed with employees annually. National Substance Abuse Recovery Month (September) is a good time for employers to affirm addiction treatment. Human resource directors and managers need to be informed about the signs of addictions in the workplace, available treatment programs, and insurance or company benefits. Allowing a negative stigma to exist regarding addiction treatment in the workplace is of no benefit to anyone. Above all, employers, managers, and supervisors need to provide reassurance that addiction treatment will be kept confidential.

Essential

Employers are beginning to recognize the high cost of addictions in the workplace. The Bureau of National Affairs has reported that chemical dependency alone costs American businesses approximately $200 billion annually. Many employers are now providing addiction treatment through health insurance, as a company benefit, and through EAPs. Some are even paying employees and providing other incentives to get treatment.

Talking to Friends and Family about Treatment

It is not easy to talk with a friend or loved one about his addiction and the need for treatment. Denial is a powerful force, certainly for the addict and often for family members and friends. The thought of facing denial may be enough to tempt one to leave the addict alone. However, remember that denial is only the outer shell of addictions. Beyond denial is an important, significant person who desperately needs help. Keep the end goal in mind as you approach this situation.

In some instances, the direct confrontational intervention approach may be helpful. However, in recent years, this has been modified and many now prefer a motivational approach to talking with a person regarding his addictions. One such approach is called CRAFT (Community Reinforcement and Family Training). The basic goal of CRAFT is to encourage loved ones to enter addiction treatment through non-confrontational methods. It promotes the use of healthy rewards to produce positive behaviors. CRAFT is directed toward both the addict and family members or loved ones. The strategies are not only designed to move the addict toward treatment, but also to enhance the quality of life for those close to the addict. Thus far, research is supporting the effectiveness of CRAFT and claims that individuals using the CRAFT method of encouraging treatment see fewer relapses than when using more direct confrontational methods. CRAFT strategies are easy to learn as well as effective.

 Alert

Addictive disorders are chronic and potentially fatal. They can ruin a person's health, social relationships, and future potential if untreated. This must be kept in mind when talking to someone submerged in addictions. Although it is the addict's responsibility to follow through with treatment and recovery, that initial confrontation may provide the necessary impetus to get her moving forward.

Getting Support

Whether you are an addict or someone close to one, support is essential. An addiction is not a solitary problem. Granted, there are those rare individuals who are able to manage addictions on their own, but the key word here is "rare." The more support one has, the more likely one can enter and maintain successful recovery. Living and/or working with an addict is not easy either. Being an encourager of an addict in treatment, sometimes having to set painful limits, can be draining. Get support! Friends, neighbors, other family members, clergy or other spiritual leaders, support groups, professional counseling, and encouraging books can all help. Don't hesitate to find supportive, trustworthy people who can maintain your confidence and offer help. Once you're in a healthier place in your life, they may gain strength from you!

CHAPTER 16

Additional Treatment Options

ADDICTIONS HAVE MULTIPLE faces and variations. A person dealing with an addiction has much in common with other addicts, yet she will also have some unique features that are hers alone. For that reason, treatments for addictions have many commonalities, but there are also treatments for those with different needs, philosophies, and lifestyles. Some of these treatments have received more support from the professional community than others. Nevertheless, the addicted person and her family can research the options, obtain professional consultation, and decide what will work best in her situation.

Detoxification

Medical stability is necessary prior to entering any type of treatment program. You will recall the significant effects and changes that drugs and alcohol have on a person's body and brain. The consequences of withdrawing from the use of drugs and alcohol can be serious and sometimes life-threatening. Safely getting drugs and/or alcohol out of a person's system is called detoxification. Detoxification is achieved by gradually reducing the dosage of the drug or by temporarily substituting another, similar drug that has less-severe side effects. During the process of detoxification, a person's vital signs (blood pressure, pulse, respiratory rate, and temperature) are monitored, emotional support is available, and medications are administered if necessary. Not everyone needs medically supervised detoxification.

An individual with a severe, longstanding addiction will likely require medical detoxification. Someone addicted to heroin, methadone, hydrocodone, OxyContin, Xanax, Vicodin, or Lortab will also require medically supervised detoxification. Other categories of individuals who should always undergo detoxification with medical supervision are the elderly, pregnant women, individuals with co-occurring psychiatric illnesses, someone who has recently consumed excessive amounts of alcohol, an addict who has no support system, and those who have previously experienced withdrawal seizures or delirium tremens.

Alert

Don't mistake detoxification for addiction treatment. Detoxification is only the beginning. It is the preparatory phase of treatment and recovery, ensuring that the addict is medically stable and able to safely engage in the treatment and recovery process. For an addict to stop treatment after detoxification is to set himself up for relapse.

The physical effects of withdrawal may include sweating, shaking, headaches, cravings, nausea, vomiting, abdominal cramps, diarrhea, loss of appetite, hyperactivity, convulsions, sleeplessness, confusion, agitation, depression, anxiety, delirium tremens, and in extreme cases, death. The effects one may experience will depend on the addictive substance and the length and quantity of use. Detoxification treatment is designed to ease the discomfort of these symptoms as much as possible. Medications may be used to relieve symptoms of detoxification. Klonopin may be used to reduce physical symptoms. Anticonvulsants such as Buprenophex and benzodiazepines to treat anxiety may also be used. Medically monitored supervision of detoxification may take three to seven days for substance addictions and three to fourteen days for alcohol addiction.

Medications Used in Addiction and Recovery

Technology has enabled scientists to gather hard evidence that addictions affect the brain. The discovery that addictions have a physiological component has led to great excitement that physiological treatments in the form of medications may be effective.

As appealing as it is to think that there are effective medical treatments for addictions, most experts agree that medications need to be used in combination with other forms of treatment such as psychotherapy. With that warning in mind, the following information about the medical treatment of addictions will provide additional hope and encouragement for those suffering with addictions.

 Fact

> The search for medical treatments for addictions is in full gear. The National Institute on Drug Abuse and the National Institute on Alcohol Abuse and Alcoholism are involved in studying more than 200 possible addiction medications. Greater understanding of how the brain operates in addictive processes has led to an explosion of treatment research.

Medications for Treating Alcohol Addiction

Acamprosate (Campral), disulfiram (Antabuse), topiramate (Topamax) and naltrexone (ReVia, Vivitrol, Depade) have all been approved by the Food and Drug Administration for treating alcohol addiction. Serzone and Zofran are two other drugs that have been found helpful in treating symptoms and complications of alcohol addiction.

- **Acamprosate (Campral)** has been available in the United States since 2004 to be used for the treatment of alcohol addiction. Campral reduces alcohol cravings and seems to work best in individuals who have already quit drinking. It may not be as effective for those who are still drinking when they start the medication or for those who are abusing other substances. Campral reduces negative feelings resulting from abstinence by stimulating GABA.

- **Disulfiram (Antabuse)** has been available since 1951. It reduces cravings and works to prevent relapse in people addicted to alcohol and cocaine. The mechanism of Antabuse is to cause the addict to feel sick if he drinks. If someone does drink while taking Antabuse, he will become flushed and develop headaches, nausea, vomiting, dizziness, and lowered blood pressure. The effects of Antabuse take place within one to two hours and are not completely out of one's system for two weeks.

- **Naltrexone (ReVia, Vivitrol, Depade)** works by blocking the parts of the brain that feel pleasure when using alcohol and narcotics. Naltrexone was originally developed to treat opiate addiction. In 1994, it was also approved for the treatment of alcoholism. Nausea is the most common side effect of naltrexone, but headaches, anxiety, dizziness, fatigue, vomiting, and insomnia may also occur. A significant problem with naltrexone has been compliance. Orally, naltrexone is taken daily and many find this bothersome over time. Long-acting naltrexone injections have recently been developed to help overcome this problem.

- **Topiramate (Topamax)** is an anticonvulsant, mood-stabilizing medication that is being investigated for use in treating alcoholism. It is thought that Topamax may reduce alcohol cravings by reducing brain levels of dopamine as well as treating the anxiety of withdrawal. Topamax has not yet been approved by the FDA for the treatment of alcoholism.

- **Nefazodone (Serzone)** is an antidepressant medication that has been found to reduce alcohol cravings. A significant side effect of Serzone is liver damage; anyone taking this medication will need to have her physician closely monitoring her liver function.

- **Ondansetron (Zofran)** has traditionally been used to treat nausea and vomiting in individuals undergoing chemotherapy. However, it has also been found to stop cravings and thus reduce alcohol consumption in early-onset alcohol addicts. The FDA is currently considering approval for this use.

 Question

What are addiction vaccines?

Addiction vaccines produce antibodies to specific drugs. The antibodies bind to the drug when it enters the bloodstream and prevent it from entering the brain. Addiction vaccines do not stop cravings nor do they treat underlying physiological problems associated with addiction. Vaccines for nicotine (NicVAX) and cocaine are currently being developed.

Medications for Treating Nicotine Addiction

Nicotine replacement products are the most popular medical treatments for nicotine addiction. They come in several forms under various brand names. Nicotine gum, nicotine patches, and nicotine lozenges may be purchased over the counter without a prescription. Nicotrol is a nasal spray that requires a prescription. These products all function by providing decreasing amounts of nicotine without smoking. Over time, the body's craving for nicotine lessens and withdrawal symptoms are eased.

Other additional medication for treating nicotine addiction include:

- **Bupropion (Zyban or Wellbutrin)** is an antidepressant medication that has demonstrated some positive benefit in helping people resist the urge to smoke. The course of treatment with bupropion begins one to two weeks prior to cessation of smoking and continues up to six months including the maintenance of smoking abstinence. Insomnia and a dry mouth are common side effects.

- **Varenicline (Chantix)** is the first medication to specifically target the neurobiological causes of nicotine dependence. It both stimulates dopamine and blocks nicotine receptors, thus reducing cravings and withdrawal symptoms. Chantix is generally prescribed for a twelve-week course of treatment. Common side effects include nausea, vomiting, gas, headaches, and insomnia.

- **Buspirone (Buspar)** and **fluoxetine (Prozac)** are additional antidepressant medications that have been successfully used to help minimize nicotine withdrawal symptoms and treat the depressive symptoms that often accompany an addiction such as nicotine.

Essential

Medications alone cannot replace or change an environment that provides triggers or encouragements to engage in addictions. Choices must still be made to avoid enticements to addictions, and this will require support and understanding from those who care about the addict and his recovery. The addicted person must not expect that medications are a cure-all for his problems.

Medications for Treating Heroin and Prescription Medication Addictions

Buprenorphine is a new medication treatment for heroin and other opiate addictions that became available in the United States in 2002. Buprenorphine is itself a narcotic and is the first narcotic that physicians can prescribe from an outpatient office setting. Although considered safer than methadone, buprenorphine itself can cause dependence and withdrawal symptoms when discontinued. Because it is prescribed on an outpatient basis, this option might not get the addict the support and mental health treatment he needs to ensure total recovery. Physicians are required to have specialized training to administer this medication.

Two forms of this drug have been approved for treatment:

- Subtex contains only buprenorphine. It is used during the first few days of treatment.
- Suboxone contains both buprenorphine and naloxone and is indicated for maintenance treatment.

Both forms of this medication come as sublingual tablets and are self-administered.

Methadone is also used to treat opiate withdrawal and has been available since the mid-1960s. It can be used to help diminish withdrawal symptoms, but is primarily used in long-term maintenance treatment. Methadone is administered daily through licensed clinics. Theoretically, an individual receiving methadone would be drug-tested to ensure abstinence from opiate use and be given psycho-social support during his clinic visit. In reality, this may or may not happen. Dependency, cognitive impairment, and depression are common side effects.

Levo-Alpha Acetyl Methadol (LAAM) is a long-acting form of methadone and an alternative to methadone treatment. It is also a replacement treatment for opiate drug addiction. LAAM requires fewer clinic visits (every two to three days), thus making it easier for a person to comply with treatment and function in a work setting.

Desipramine (Norpramin) is an antidepressant that has been found to be helpful in treating individuals with opiate addictions and encouraging abstinence.

Medications for Treating Cocaine Addiction

Several medications are now available to help in the treatment of cocaine addiction. In general, they focus on reducing cravings for cocaine and blocking the euphoric effects of cocaine.

- **Baclofen** is a muscle relaxant that has primarily been used to treat muscle spasms in individuals suffering from multiple sclerosis. It has recently been demonstrated that baclofen also reduces cravings in cocaine addicts. Baclofen achieves this effect by inhibiting the release of dopamine in the brain and also by increasing the amount of GABA available to the brain. This medication is especially helpful for addicts who have been chronic, heavy users of cocaine. Typical side effects of baclofen include drowsiness, weakness, fatigue, and nausea.
- **Gabapentin (Gabitrol)** is another anticonvulsant medication that has been found to reduce cravings for cocaine and seems to lessen the severity of relapses. Gabitrol works by increasing GABA in the brain. Sedation is the primary side effect.
- **Gamma-vinyl-GABA (GVG)** or vigabatrin is an antiepileptic medication that may reduce cocaine cravings as well as cravings for inhalants, heroin, and nicotine. This medication also works to increase the amount of GABA in the brain. Sleepiness and fatigue are typical side effects. This medication is not yet available in the United States.
- **Nocaine** is a weaker version of cocaine. As a treatment for cocaine addiction, it blocks the stimulant effects of cocaine. At this time, one may only obtain this medication by participating in clinical research trials. Side effects are unknown.
- **Modafinil (Provigil)** is a medication that tends to reduce the "high" sensation caused by cocaine. It also helps diminish cocaine cravings. The exact mechanism of Provigil is unknown, other than it does increase glutamate in the brain. Typical side effects include headaches, back pain, nausea, nervousness, insomnia, and anxiety. Provigil also carries with it the risk of dependency.

Miscellaneous Medication Information

Medications can certainly give the addict the boost she needs to help in addiction recovery. Amazing research on addiction medications is in progress, and it has been said that in ten years, the whole landscape of medical addiction treatment will be changed. In the meantime, as wonderful as medication advances and treatments are, the recovering addict must be careful. Over-the-counter medications taken for other ailments—such as cough syrups, mouthwashes, antihistamines, cold and sinus medications, pain relievers, nasal sprays, decongestants, and prescription medications for other medical disorders—may affect receptor areas in the brain that could trigger cravings, leading to a relapse. A recovering addict must always let his prescribing physician know about his situation so that wise medication choices can be made.

Alternative Treatment Options

Not everyone subscribes to traditional and medical treatments for addictions. Individuals from different cultures and different spiritual faiths may have particular reasons to pursue alternative treatments. For some, natural and holistic approaches to health care are very important philosophically.

 Question

What are "yin," "yang," and "qi"?
Yin and yang are opposing forces in nature and must be in balance for health and well-being. Concepts associated with yin include negatives, shade, female, cold, inner, and upper. Those associated with yang include positives, bright, male, heat, outer, and lower. Qi is the vital energy flowing throughout one's body, bringing nourishment to body tissues and promoting healthy functioning of internal organs.

Biofeedback

Biofeedback is a scientific method of treatment using monitors to provide a person physiological feedback. In the 1950s and 1960s, Neal E. Miller, an experimental psychologist, proposed that a person could be trained to control her autonomic, or involuntary, nervous system. By watching physiological (respiration, blood pressure, temperature, etc.) feedback on the monitor, a person can adjust her thinking patterns to control her body. This was a controversial idea in the beginning, but time has demonstrated this technique to be effective in treating numerous conditions, including addictions.

Biofeedback helps treat addictions in two ways. First, it trains a person to decrease his anxiety levels. High anxiety is related to increased drug withdrawal severity and lower tolerance for withdrawal symptoms. Second, brain wave biofeedback (or neurofeedback) helps someone learn to alter his brain wave patterns. Alpha and theta brain waves are disturbed with long-term substance addiction. Brain wave biofeedback can train a person to normalize these brain waves, resulting in prevention of relapses.

Acupuncture

Acupuncture is a form of traditional Chinese medicine developed thousands of years ago. Its effectiveness was recognized by the FDA in March 1996, when acupuncture was approved as a medical treatment in the United States.

Acupuncture entails the insertion of very fine needles plus the application of heat or electrical stimuli into specified acupuncture channels throughout the body. Chinese medical theory proposes that all diseases are caused by disturbances in one's yin, yang, qi (or chi), and blood. The purpose of acupuncture is to adjust and correct these forces and bring them into balance. In treating addictions, acupuncture reportedly raises endorphin levels, helping an addict to control cravings and withdrawal symptoms such as nausea and the "shakes." Acupuncture has been used in all stages of addiction to treat barbiturate, cocaine, nicotine, heroin, alcohol, and other addictions with no known side effects. Acupuncture advocates claim that this treatment can help a person maintain abstinence by treating the underlying stress that may have contributed to the development of the addiction.

Hypnosis

Hypnosis involves being in a state of focused concentration and relaxation. A hypnotized person is in a trancelike state that enables her to be susceptible to therapeutic suggestions provided by the hypnotherapist. It is unknown exactly how hypnosis works. Some believe it causes the brain to release natural substances such as endorphins that affect the way one perceives symptoms such as pain. Others believe that hypnosis helps a person to unconsciously control physiological reactions such as blood pressure, heart rate, hunger, and so forth. Hypnosis has been used in the treatment of many disorders and was recognized in 1958 by the American Medical Association as a valid medical treatment. Its primary use in treating addictions has been to help with smoking cessation, although it has also been used to treat addictions to alcohol, other drugs, and food. Some believe that hypnosis does not provide long-term addiction recovery but only temporary and superficial relief. Many misconceptions exist pertaining to hypnosis, but the truth is that:

- Hypnosis is not a state of sleep.
- The hypnotized person is quite able to control his behavior during hypnosis and is very aware of his surroundings.
- Hypnosis does not increase the accuracy of one's memory.
- Amnesia after being hypnotized is quite rare.
- A hypnotized person cannot be forced through suggestion to engage in any activity he feels is wrong.

It is important to know that there are no formal licensing requirements in the United States for hypnotherapists. Therefore, it is very important to research the training, experience, and professional reputation of the hypnotherapist one chooses to use for treatment.

Aromatherapy

Aromatherapy is the use of essential oils derived from plants and herbs. These oils are either inhaled or applied topically to the skin. The theory behind aromatherapy is that herbaceous essential oils contain naturally occurring chemicals that promote emotional balance, relieve stress, and calm one's spirit. Aromatherapy is related to flower essence therapy. They differ in that flower essences are likened more to homeopathy, a dilution of the flower essence. Proponents of these types of therapies claim that traditional biomedical treatments for addictions deny the impact of the spirit and soul in healing. Aromatherapy and flower essence therapies promote a spiritual healing that enhances long-term recovery.

 Fact

> The placebo effect is a phenomenon whereby a "fake" treatment with an inactive substance, such as sugar or a saline solution, leads to improvement in a person's health simply because the person expects that to happen. The greater the expectation that the person will benefit from the "treatment," the more likely that is to happen.

Homeopathy

Homeopathy is a type of natural medicine that uses extremely diluted amounts of substances that might actually produce symptoms of the disease being treated if administered in the original concentration. Homeopathic remedies are derived from plants, minerals, and animal sources. The basic theory of homeopathy is that "like cures like." Homeopathy doesn't claim to treat chemical dependencies per se. However, it does purport to treat the causes and consequences of addictions, such as pain, anxiety, depression, and restlessness.

Tuberculinum, argentum, nitricum, arsenicum, and other substances are commonly used in treating the effects of addictions. As with other holistic approaches to treatment, the goal of homeopathy is to restore the body's natural balance. The effectiveness of homeopathy is controversial. Critics say homeopathy works because of a placebo effect and has no real medicinal value.

Herbal Therapy

Herbs are natural plant substances that have effects on physiological functioning. Herbology is the use of herbs to treat illness, including addictions. Herbs as adjuncts to treating addiction primarily help in detoxification and treating symptoms that make for a more comfortable withdrawal period. Strengthening the body with herbal treatments during recovery may promote prevention of relapse. Common herbs used to detoxify and strengthen the liver include milk thistle, goldenseal, dandelion, bupleurum, skullcap, valerian, passionflower, chamomile, and ginkgo. Herbs that may strengthen the immune system include Siberian ginseng, American ginseng, and astragalus. These are just some examples; many more herbs have been suggested as helping in the treatment of addictions. One should consult a knowledgeable herbologist to find the right combination of herbs that may be helpful in treating a person's particular symptoms.

Wisdom dictates that one should consider the following guidelines in using herbs:

- Do not use unidentified herbs.
- Do not use narcotic herbs or plants.
- Use only recommended dosages of herbs.
- Use mildly toxic herbs, such as belladonna, only under a physician's supervision.
- Do not take combinations of herbs at the same time without professional supervision.
- If an extreme physical reaction occurs as the result of taking herbs, contact one's physician immediately or go to the nearest emergency room.

Nutrition

Drug and alcohol addictions are notorious for leading to malnutrition and chemical imbalances in one's body. Nutritional therapy in the treatment of addictions is designed to restore the body's balance of amino acids, essential fatty acids, vitamins, and minerals. The body requires proper nutrition to enable it to naturally produce neurotransmitters such as norepinephrine, serotonin, and endorphins. Throughout this book, it has been emphasized how important these chemicals are in the regulation of mood and behavior. The amino acid tyrosine is a precursor needed for the production of norepinephrine and the amino acid tryptophan is a precursor needed for the production of serotonin. Vitamin C is often helpful to moderate physical and emotional symptoms of withdrawal and detoxification.

Hypoglycemia, or low blood sugar, often develops in alcoholics, and amphetamine and heroin addicts and may cause depression, anxiety, panic attacks, and mood swings. This condition may be treated by a professional with nutrients such as niacin, chromium, and magnesium after detoxification. Nutrients that are beneficial in detoxifying and strengthening the liver and digestive tract include Vitamin C, selenium, zinc, chromium, and acidophilus. Calcium, magnesium, and DL-phenylalanine relax and strengthen the nervous system. The B vitamins are often deficient in individuals who have used excessive amounts of sugar, caffeine, alcohol, or other drugs. Potassium deficiencies are also common. A healthy, well-rounded diet of fresh fruits and vegetables, carbohydrates, and quality proteins is always a good idea. To get started on the path to healthy nutrition when recovering from addictions, it is quite helpful to consult with a nutritionist who specializes in working with recovering addicts.

Meditation, Guided Imagery, and Yoga

Meditation is often combined with deep breathing practices and is intended to help a person quiet her mind. The purpose of meditation is to create an environment of peacefulness and quiet that allows one to get in touch with the soul and spirit. Guided imagery is different in that there is a specific focus that a person dwells on to achieve peacefulness.

Yoga is a technique that uses various physical postures and controlled breathing to increase flexibility, calm the mind, improve concentration and focus, and build patience. These therapies are very helpful adjuncts for an addict dealing with the stress of detoxification, withdrawal, and recovery.

Creative Arts Therapies

What are creative arts therapies? Dance, music, drama, poetry, writing, movement, and visual arts such as painting, coloring, and ceramics are the most common examples of creative arts therapies. Many addiction treatment programs, both inpatient and outpatient, incorporate some or all of these therapies as enhancements to other forms of treatment. Creative arts therapies serve many valuable purposes in treating addictions. First, they provide a relaxed atmosphere in which someone can reconnect with his inner self, begin to define himself in a healthier manner, and get in touch with his spirituality. Creative arts therapies allow an individual to express difficult and painful emotions in a variety of ways. Not everyone is comfortable expressing these situations verbally. Someone who has been mired in an addictive lifestyle may be out of the habit of enjoying life, and creative arts therapies can help.

 Question

What is Ayurveda?
Ayurveda is a natural system of medicine that has been practiced in India for over 5,000 years. Ayurveda is based on the belief that all disease begins with an imbalance or stress in a person's consciousness. Lifestyle interventions and natural therapies are used to prevent and treat diseases.

Outdoor Therapy

Outdoor therapy uses experiences in nature to assist an addict struggling to achieve a sober and healthy lifestyle. Backpacking, white-water rafting, rock climbing, and learning survival skills are coordinated to help the addict develop self-confidence, responsibility, social skills, and a healthy lifestyle of exercise and nutrition.

Trained addiction counselors accompany the group into a nature setting, providing individual and group counseling as part of the program. These programs often last three to six weeks and may be covered by insurance if they are accredited. Both adult and adolescent programs have been developed.

Self-Help Options

Many of the treatment options outlined in this chapter may be done on a self-help basis. An initial consultation with a professional to get one started may be helpful and encourage confidence that the addict can indeed do things to promote her own recovery. Certainly, educating herself by reading informative material in books, the Internet, and professional journals will prepare a person to understand and implement what is needed for recovery. Taking the initiative to join a support group can help one to develop a sense of camaraderie in this process. Online support groups are also becoming quite popular and have the advantage of being available twenty-four hours a day, seven days a week.

 Fact

Animal or pet therapy is yet another alternative form of treatment for recovering addicts. Interacting with animals tends to lower one's heart rate and blood pressure, increase endorphin levels, decrease stress levels, and provide a sense of calm well-being. Equine therapy in particular is a well-established form of outdoor experiential therapy.

Faith-Based Treatment Programs

Faith-based treatment programs began over seventy years ago with Alcoholics Anonymous and its Twelve-Step program of recovery based on a "Higher Power."

Studies have shown that among individuals in recovery, higher levels of religious faith and spirituality correlated positively with optimism, greater perceived social support, lower levels of anxiety, and greater resilience in stressful situations. People with religious faith have also been shown to be less likely to be addicted to drugs and alcohol. The government has taken note and joined forces with faith-based addiction treatment programs. In 2000, the U.S. Substance Abuse and Mental Health Services Administration (SAMHSA) became the first federal agency through the U.S. Department of Health and Human Services to become involved with the Faith-Based and Community Initiatives. Currently, one-third of federal vouchers made available through the Access to Recovery (ATR) Program have been paid to faith-based treatment programs.

Essential

All major faiths have developed organized addiction treatment programs—Christian, Jewish, Muslim, Buddhist, and Hindu. Religious faith has been a source of support and encouragement to people struggling with addictions for many years. Many people find that religious faith provides hope that an addict can achieve the healthy lifestyle that he seeks.

The Risks of Treatment

The risks of treatment apply to all forms of treatment, whether conventional or alternative. Medication side effects and side effects of herbal and nutritional supplements must be considered. One must also consider the risk of placing one's treatment in the hands of a professional with inadequate training. There is the risk of losing friends and family members who are not ready to give up their addictions. Going into treatment may cost someone his job or cause a setback in his academic courses. There is certainly the risk of financial setbacks because of the cost of treatment. However, the greatest risk of all is getting no treatment. All the risks of treatment can be successfully managed with education, consultation with qualified professionals, and belief in one's ability to achieve recovery. The hard work and sacrifices will be worth it!

CHAPTER 17

Recovery

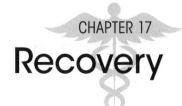

THERE ARE NO known cures for addictions. Nevertheless, a person can overcome addictions and learn to manage life successfully. Many tools are available to help with this process. The most important tool is found within oneself—the desire to overcome addiction and adopt a healthier lifestyle. Although initially this desire may be weak and even born out of wanting to avoid negative consequences, it's a start. With support and knowledge, recovery is achievable. A healthy future is within reach!

Become Knowledgeable about Recovery

As shown in Chapter 16, there are many approaches to accomplishing recovery. In choosing a route to recovery, one must consider the primary addiction, complicating co-occurring addictions and/or physical health problems, the possible presence of co-occurring mental health disorders, one's philosophy of treatment, the availability of resources, cultural and ethnic influences, and available support networks. Once a person has done his homework and decided on a course to recovery, it's time to get started. Recovery occurs in three phases:

- **Phase One** is making a commitment to recovery, detoxification, and stabilizing one's physical health.
- **Phase Two** involves making changes to achieve a lifestyle of recovery and repairing physical, emotional, spiritual, and relational damages caused by the addiction.
- **Phase Three** is maintenance and a commitment with a plan to never return to a life ruled by addictions.

Many an individual finds that she is grateful for the addiction in the end. Initially, that may sound very strange. However, the process of recovery can lead a person to a place of honesty, health, and inner peace that she would never have reached had she not been faced with the challenge of dealing with an addiction. Thinking of recovery as an opportunity is a first step in working with the process.

L, Essential

Recovery from addictions is not just stopping the use of the addictive substance and/or behavior. If underlying thought patterns, problematic relationships, and dysfunctional behaviors aren't changed, relapse is inevitable. Addictions are powerful forces and must be battled on multiple fronts to reach lasting recovery.

Changing Thinking Patterns

Cognitive-behavioral therapy (CBT) is one of the most common and successfully used therapeutic methods for treating addictions. CBT is based on the premise that dysfunctional beliefs lead to forming unrealistic expectations and negative thought patterns. Unrealistic expectations and negative thought patterns then lead to painful emotions and problematic behaviors. These dysfunctional beliefs, unrealistic expectations, and negative thought patterns are typically based on lies, assumptions, and distortions that the addict has accepted as true.

Lying is often an essential part of addictions. One lies about using the substance or engaging in the behavior, lies about the consequences incurred as a result of the addiction, and lies to maintain a façade of respectability. Honesty and truth are foundational components of successful recovery. This means that thinking patterns and beliefs must change to reflect truthfulness. What are some of the common dysfunctional thoughts and beliefs about addictions? Here are some examples:

- The addiction is not my fault.
- The addiction is the only way I can cope with my painful emotions.
- The addiction enhances my creativity and performance.
- The addiction enables me to fit in socially.
- The addiction is not a problem.
- The addiction is a character flaw and I don't deserve to recover.
- Using is fun, not using is boring.
- I need the addiction to relax.
- The addiction is in control and is stronger than I am.

 Question

What is cognitive-behavioral therapy (CBT)?
CBT was developed by Aaron T. Beck in the early 1990s. It is a short-term, focused approach to treatment that involves both functional analysis and skills training. Negative beliefs and thought patterns, which result in uncomfortable emotions and dysfunctional behaviors, are addressed. Coping and change strategies help the addict make rational, healthy choices.

One can see that as long as these notions are entertained as true, it will be very difficult to engage in successful recovery. How does CBT help with changing dysfunctional thinking? There are several techniques that may be helpful when used appropriately by a professional trained in CBT. One technique is asking leading questions that challenge dysfunctional, negative beliefs and thoughts. Addicts commonly adopt thinking patterns that reflect an "all-or-nothing" or "black-or-white" perspective. These perspectives are seldom accurate and need to be challenged.

A CBT therapist may also have the addict analyze the advantages and disadvantages of the addiction, encouraging logical re-evaluation of the addiction. Identification of dysfunctional beliefs is key to successful change. These beliefs must be reformulated to become accurate and honest. Another technique of CBT is helping the addict reassign responsibility for the addictions. An addict will frequently blame people and circumstances outside of himself for his addiction. Until the addict can recognize his internal motivations for the addictions, he will be unable to modify his own addictive behaviors. Guided imagery and role-playing are techniques designed to help the addict visualize himself avoiding the addiction and making healthy choices. Rehearsal is a technique that helps the addict cognitively practice healthy, honest thoughts and beliefs about his addiction. Here are some examples:

- I don't have to lie about my addiction.
- I will feel better physically without my addiction.
- I can accomplish more of my goals without my addiction.
- I can have better relationships without my addiction.
- I will be better off financially without my addiction.
- I can think more clearly when not focused on my addiction.
- I will have more time to pursue hobbies and interests when not involved with my addiction.
- I will have more self-confidence when I've overcome my addiction.
- I will not have to worry about getting into trouble with the law when I'm no longer involved with my addiction.

Healthy behaviors are more likely to follow accurate, positive, goal-oriented thoughts. While initially CBT may focus primarily on developing control of the addiction, subsequent CBT therapy will focus on the development of skills that will result in a lifetime of healthy recovery.

Cognitive-behavioral therapy alone may not be enough to promote healthy recovery. Medications, group support, and other treatment modalities may also be necessary. This is especially true if addictions are complicated with co-occurring mental health or physical problems. The good news is that CBT is highly effective used in conjunction with other therapies.

Fact

Daily thought records (DTRs) are often used by CBT therapists in treating an addicted person. This is a type of homework assignment completed by the addict with the purpose of helping her to analyze and change her thinking patterns. The addict is to write about situations, automatic thoughts, emotions, rational responses, and outcomes related to troubling moods and circumstances.

Technological Aids

Technology is bringing new help to those in recovery. It is making support and knowledge available to a wider audience than ever before. Another advantage of technological help is its constant availability—around the clock, seven days a week. What are some of these aids? The computer, of course, is a primary one. Internet radio programs such as *www.recoveryradio.net/index2.html* broadcast around the clock. They provide twelve-step speakers, addiction recovery news, information about addictions, workshops, and opportunities to chat with others in recovery. The shows at Take 12 Radio (*http://khlt .homestead.com/home.html*) focus on the twelve-step approach to recovery and relapse prevention. Talk programs plus music promoting recovery are featured. Recovery Coast to Coast (*http://recovery coasttocoast.org*) is a talk show available nightly. It is sponsored by the Alliance for Recovery and features interviews, testimonials from people in recovery, and call-ins from listeners.

Multiple online message boards and chat rooms are available for twelve-step meetings of all kinds. Sites are available for addicts as well as family members. While going to actual meetings may provide a needed personal connection, if an addict is ill, has no transportation, or is simply not ready, he doesn't have to miss a meeting as online meetings are available on a regular basis. There are also free online movies and television programs available through *www.sobriety.tv*. The programs at this site provide information about addiction recovery, help with the twelve steps, personal recovery stories, and much more. Home Box Office (HBO) has completed a major documentary covering several different components of addiction that can be viewed online as well (*www.hbo.com/addiction/thefilm/index.html?current=5*).

Essential

> Technology is within one's control. It can be a source of addictions or a source of treatment and support. If technology has previously fed into one's addictions, place blocks on the sites of concern. Learning to use technology in a positive manner to enhance recovery may be one more benefit of reprogramming one's thinking and associations.

Of course, there are unlimited articles, research, and information pieces regarding addictions and recovery available on the Internet. Although it is impossible to list all of these sites, some significant ones are listed in Appendix A. Hand-held computers that are now found in combination with cellular phones and other hand-held devices make it more convenient than ever to complete therapeutic homework such as recording thoughts, triggers, feelings, and so forth.

One can even provide support and encouragement to someone struggling with addictions through an e-card. Free e-cards designed to inspire recovery can be accessed at: *www.123greetings.com /encouragement_and_inspiration/health*. It seems there is no end to the possibilities of technology in aiding addiction recovery. Technology addicts, however, may want to use caution and utilize other types of addiction recovery aids.

Question

What is telemedicine?
Telemedicine is the use of video and/or computer technology to access mental health care from rural or remote areas. A person can speak with a health care provider and, if video components are available, the provider can also observe the person calling. This technology can also be used among professionals for consultations and training purposes.

Avoiding Relapse

As simple as it sounds, the first step to avoiding relapse for the recovering addict is to identify what is tempting. Temptations put one in a high-risk situation for relapse. Temptations tend to remind a person of the "good times" associated with addictions. When temptations present themselves, the addict often seems to develop selective amnesia about the inevitable negative consequences. Temptations are dependent on the strength of the desire or the inclination to partake of the addiction. They are closely tied to how one feels about oneself. An individual with a strong sense of self and purpose will be much more able to withstand temptations. A person with low self-esteem who is struggling with painful emotions will be more susceptible to giving in to temptation, and thus relapse. Temptations leading to relapse tend to be associated with places where activities surrounding the addiction took place, people associated with the addiction, and tangible and intangible "things" associated with the addiction. Avoiding temptation, and thereby preventing relapse, means recognizing the associations, acknowledging their power to draw one in again, and giving them a wide berth.

Addictions typically become connected with certain patterns, rituals, and people. Here are examples of some temptations that might lead one to relapse:

- Nostalgic music that may be associated with the addiction.
- White, powdery kitchen items such as flour, sugar, baking powder, baking soda, and cornstarch may resemble cocaine.
- Television programs and movies may have scenes that remind one of using days.
- A particular intersection may remind one of meeting a dealer.
- The hours of four to six in the evening may be associated with cocktails after work.
- Developing a respiratory infection or a headache may remind one of prescription drugs used in an addictive manner.
- Running into a using "buddy" at the shopping mall may unexpectedly bring to mind one's addiction.

 Fact

Temptations are harder to resist at certain times. Alcoholics Anonymous uses the acronym HALT to remind us of the times when temptations are most appealing. When someone is Hungry, Angry, Lonely, and/or Tired, danger of relapse is ahead. In recognizing these situations, a person can take pre-emptive action and protect her recovery.

Each recovering addict will have his own peculiar associations with his addictions. Taking steps to prevent temptation, and thus relapse, from arising is the best approach to protecting one's recovery. Clean out anything in the medicine cabinet that may relate to prescription drug use. Remove alcohol from the liquor cabinet. Place filters and blocks on one's computer and place the computer in a common family area. Don't go alone to locations where known temptations wait.

Be careful of hidden temptations as well. One's best efforts and intentions may be sabotaged by temptations that seemingly come out of nowhere. Unasked for pop-ups may appear on one's computer screen tempting one to re-enter pornographic sites. Going to a fine restaurant for an enjoyable meal may stimulate old temptations after tasting foods cooked with alcohol. The innocent sound of cooking spray used before scrambling breakfast eggs may bring back memories of inhalant use. Beware of jokes about past addictions. Although the intent may be to lighten one's mood, the reminder may bring heavy temptation to the forefront of the addict's mind. The good news is that the more often one successfully wards off temptations, the weaker they become. As the recovering addict recognizes her ability to manage temptation, her confidence gains strength and lifelong recovery is within her grasp.

Alert

Smell, taste, touch, hearing, and sight are all avenues whereby temptations can connect. The smell of certain foods may tempt a food addict, the taste of alcohol may tempt the alcoholic, touching certain objects may tempt the shoplifter, hearing the roll of dice may tempt the gambling addict, and seeing a certain advertisement might tempt one to smoke. Be aware and thus be prepared!

Effective Use of Support Systems

Several references have already been made regarding support systems. However, developing a solid and lifelong recovery from addictions may require regular evaluations of one's support systems and their effectiveness. This requires a proactive approach by the recovering addict. There are many situations in which adjustments to one's support systems might be appropriate.

Once a person has completed detoxification, has made significant changes in lifestyle, and is well into recovery, her needs may change. She may have outgrown her initial support system in knowledge and experience. Either the addict will need to encourage her support system to become more educated about more advanced recovery as well, or she will need to seek out supportive people with knowledge matching her level of recovery.

One of the greatest dangers for the addict in recovery is boredom, including boredom with support systems. For example, a recovering alcoholic may become bored with A.A., saying he's heard the same messages over and over again. Nothing is new. How does one deal with this? A recovering addict needs to take the initiative to create his own interest. Using the A.A. example, he can go to different meetings and become acquainted with new people, he can volunteer to lead the meeting and introduce topics of interest, or he can invite A.A. friends to socialize outside of meetings. Heading the start-up of a new support group can be an exciting challenge and there's nothing like passing on what one has learned to develop positive feelings about oneself.

 Question

How can a recovering addict expand her support system to meet ever-changing needs?
Apathy and boredom are common problems for longtime recovering addicts. A recovering addict needs to challenge himself and also have a challenging support system. Becoming involved in regional and/or national recovery groups may be just the thing to bring new purpose and meaning to recovery. Working with others to develop new programs for addicts just entering recovery may also be quite stimulating.

Another danger for a recovering addict is thinking he's beaten the addiction and no longer needs support. This is dangerous territory. Often this indicates that old patterns of negative thinking and dysfunctional behaviors may still be lurking in the shadows of one's mind. An effective support system is made of individuals who will not be afraid to challenge the recovering addict to re-examine his thought processes. It is very important that a recovering addict choose a support system with individuals who will be honest even when he doesn't like what they have to say. Finally, lacking direction and/or purpose in one's life is also a threat to long-lasting recovery. Effective use of one's support system may include getting new ideas and perspectives from people in different walks of life. Having trustworthy people with whom to explore life's issues and bounce ideas around may be exactly what's needed to keep forward movement in recovery going.

Essential

Getting too comfortable with recovery is dangerous. Becoming overconfident, passive, and relaxed can set a person up for self-sabotage and relapse. Developing an active support system that is adaptable to one's needs and level of recovery is essential for maintenance of a healthy lifestyle.

Utilizing Community Resources

For the person in recovery, community resources can be a gateway to supporting an addiction-free lifestyle. Support groups such as Alcoholics Anonymous, Narcotics Anonymous, and other twelve-step groups have already been mentioned but deserve mention again as they contribute so much to the lives of recovering addicts.

There are many other community resources that also promote a healthy, addiction-free life. The YMCA offers opportunities for exercise, classes to learn new skills, and social events to promote healthy socialization in the community. Many communities offer adult community education programs where a person can explore new interests and develop new skills. These classes may lead to a new career or may simply stimulate one's mind, simultaneously developing new friends. Many churches, synagogues, and other religious institutions have programs supporting sobriety and recovery. They provide excellent opportunities for the recovering addict to heal and grow spiritually. Religious organizations also provide additional opportunities to meet other individuals who are more likely to be committed to a sober lifestyle.

Additionally, most communities have various clubs and organizations devoted to particular interests. Examples include golf clubs, garden clubs, book clubs, bridge clubs, and dance clubs. While these community activities may not be specifically for supporting addiction recovery, they do promote the development of hobbies and interests that fit in with a healthy, addiction-free life.

Alert

In spite of vast educational and awareness efforts, there may still be those in communities who retain prejudices against recovering addicts. Some may hold on to fears relating addictions to crime and family pain. Don't let the prejudices and fears of others stand in the way of recovery! Be prepared, and in spite of these barriers, live an exemplary life devoted to recovery.

Last, but not least, are community political organizations. These groups provide excellent opportunities for a recovering addict to contribute to building healthy communities for himself and others alike. Working to enact ordinances and laws affecting addiction recovery in one's community can boost a sense of self-worth and accomplishment.

The Face of Healthy Recovery

Healthy recovery is a multifaceted process. It involves a commitment to change, leaving behind the attachments of addictions. Indeed, change from a life of addictions can be fearful. The first change to be made, therefore, is how one approaches recovery. It must be seen as an opportunity and a great adventure! Healthy recovery encompasses every aspect of one's life. Physical health requires exercise, well-rounded nutrition, and maintenance of a healthy weight. Emotional and psychological health involves learning to manage one's emotions appropriately and developing a sense of peace and contentment with one's place in life. Social health is the task of developing loyal, honest, and deep family relationships and friendships as well as learning to comfortably interact with strangers and acquaintances. Spiritual health is examining one's spiritual beliefs and developing depth in that area. Occupational health is discovering one's interests, talents, and skills, then utilizing that combination to find a rewarding way in which to earn a living. The face of healthy recovery is a lifetime of learning about one's identity and place in the world. It can provide a sense of euphoria with which no addiction can compare!

CHAPTER 18

Relapse Prevention

RECOVERY FROM ADDICTIONS is a major accomplishment. It takes tremendous commitment and hard work. Courage is required to face the dark side of an addiction, admit to the damage it's caused, and risk trying healthier behaviors. The healthier behaviors of recovery may initially feel strange, unfamiliar, and frightening. Therefore, needless to say, recovery is the victory of a very hard-fought battle. The last thing one wants to consider is relapse. Nevertheless, relapse is a possibility every recovering addict must acknowledge. The best defense against relapse is preparation and prevention.

Be Prepared

The first six months of abstaining from an addiction are the most difficult. During these six months, most of the typical temptations, triggers, and challenges will occur at some point. If someone can successfully cope with these problems and maintain abstinence, then some stability will be established and recovery will begin to get easier. Therefore, be prepared to endure. Recovery will not happen overnight. How can a person prepare for successful recovery? As with any battle, it is essential to know as much as possible about one's enemy—in this case, relapse.

What are the most common causes of relapse?

- Continually berating oneself for having an addiction.
- Preoccupation with the past, including the pleasures associated with one's addiction.
- Hanging on to guilt and shame over the addiction.

- Persistent blaming of oneself or others for the problems caused by addiction.
- Overconfidence with one's initial abstinence.
- Self-centeredness and self-pity related to the addiction.
- Negative thinking or the fear of trusting any successes.
- Sampling of the addictive substance or behavior. This may happen inadvertently, such as tasting food cooked in alcohol.

The common denominator of these causes of relapse is having one foot in the addictive past. Successful recovery requires a forward focus. One must deal with the past, acknowledging and taking responsibility for wrongs done to others out of one's addictions, making amends if possible, and managing the consequences of addictions as positively as one can. Old, dysfunctional thought patterns and behaviors must be transformed into ones that are true, productive, and healthy. Once those things are accomplished, it's time to move on. Recovery is a word associated with the future, not the past.

 Question

How common is it for a recovering addict to relapse?
The National Institute on Drug Abuse (NIDA) states that the relapse rates for recovering addicts (40 to 60 percent) are similar to those for individuals managing chronic diseases such as diabetes (30 to 50 percent), hypertension (50 to 70 percent), and asthma (50 to 70 percent). Ninety percent of recovering addicts will have a brief period of relapse. The majority of these brief relapses occur within the first month of recovery.

One activity that many have found helpful in being prepared is the "what if" exercise. This exercise works best with someone who knows the recovering addict well and who will be willing to role-play responses. All possible scenarios that might set off a slip or relapse are brought up for discussion. The recovering addict then brainstorms how he might handle each situation to avoid relapse. Here are some examples:

- What if an old friend the addict used with calls and wants to get together?
- What if the alcoholic finds a hidden bottle of vodka that she missed when she was cleaning her house of alcohol?
- What if a friend invites the pornography addict to an "R-rated" movie with sexually explicit scenes?
- What if a food addict is invited to a birthday party where his favorite cake is being served?
- What if a gambling addict is invited to participate in a Vegas-style fundraiser?
- What if a nicotine addict is invited to a family function where everyone else is smoking and she knows she'll be offered a cigarette to be sociable?

With potential responses already in mind and practiced, it's much easier to handle these tempting and difficult situations.

 Fact

Brain-imaging studies have demonstrated the struggle to avoid relapse. Visual cues as short as thirty-three milliseconds that are related to one's substance abuse can activate the dopamine reward circuit. This process begins before conscious awareness. Once this occurs, the decision-making functions of the brain's frontal lobe become less effective. The result is greater difficulty in resisting the urge to relapse.

Another suggestion is to always have a "plan of escape." When it seems impossible to avoid problematic situations, maybe because of family obligations or work requirements, have a logical, but honest, rationale for needing to leave the scene if the temptations become too strong. Take a separate means of transportation, if necessary, so that dependence on another person for a ride will not be a hindrance to leaving a stressful situation. This is no reason to feel guilty; protecting one's recovery is saving one's life.

Alert

Adolescents are at particularly high risk for addiction relapse. This is partly due to their developmental stage in life. The immature brains of adolescents are often disposed to poor decision-making and lack of impulse control. Adolescents with the additional risk factors of learning disabilities, dysfunctional family systems, and/or a dual diagnosis need extra help in maintaining recovery.

Since there may be times when triggers and temptations are unavoidable, another strategy to manage these times is to condition oneself to have a different response to the temptation. Professional therapeutic help may be required to accomplish this. Desensitization, relaxation training, distractions, and positive self-talk are all methods one can use to retrain the response to an addictive cue. For example, learning relaxation training in order to get in a relaxed state prior to encountering an addictive cue can help one replace feelings of excitement with feelings of calm and indifference. A person addicted to pornography will need to learn the skill of distraction if he's ever to go to the beach again on vacation. He will need to learn to refocus his attention to the sea life, to learning scuba diving, and to the wonderful taste of fresh lobster. Although this may seem too difficult, it most definitely can be accomplished with help from a professional.

Learning the art of positive self-talk is an essential skill for a recovering addict. Saying to oneself, "I can focus much better on the conversation with a glass of iced tea than with a martini" or "I am more than able to use my creativity to come up with new outfits from my own closet. I don't need to spend more to look good" are just two examples of positive self-talk. It's a good idea to develop a list of positive self-talk statements to have handy whenever recovery is threatened. Reviewing these statements daily is also a great preventative measure to avoid slips and relapse.

Recognizing Triggers

Triggers have many similarities to temptations, but may be more subtle. Triggers may be thought of as preludes to temptations. They may be so closely tied together that no distinction is noticeable. Triggers bring to life the awareness of a connection between feelings, places, people, things, or situations and cravings for one's addiction. Loneliness may trigger one's craving for the social chaos of a gambling casino. Depression may trigger one's craving for a plate of double fudge brownies. Anger may trigger a craving for the calming effect of Xanax. Marital discord may trigger the craving to escape into the sexual world of the Internet. Driving by one's old high school football stadium may trigger memories of drinking with friends, thus reviving a craving for alcohol.

Essential

A recovering addict who has gone through inpatient or partial hospitalization treatment will have received help to develop an aftercare plan. Someone in outpatient treatment, or recovering on her own, can also develop an aftercare plan. Essentially, this is a plan of action, written down, that describes supports to use, coping strategies, and people to call for help when needed.

Triggers are the threshold to relapse and addiction. Triggers cannot be ignored if a recovering addict is to remain in recovery.

Knowing one's weaknesses is the first step to being prepared with a strategy for successfully overcoming them.

Managing—and Recovering from—Slips

Slips are a prelude to relapse. A slip is that one drink, that one piece of chocolate, or that one peek at pornography. It's a one-time mistake. Relapse is a falling away from the pattern of recovery. It is taking one "slip" and multiplying it into many that last days, weeks, months, or years. Relapse, simply put, is turning back to one's addiction and, once again, embracing the addictive lifestyle. The way a person manages a slip, the way she thinks about a slip, may well determine whether the slip stays a mistake or whether it progresses to relapse. The recovering addict must guard his thoughts carefully when it comes to a slip. He must remind himself that the thought of a slip is only a close call, an actual slip is only a mistake. Allowing this to go further and thinking of oneself as a failure because of a slip is to head full-speed toward relapse.

If the recovering addict can think of a slip as a learning experience rather than a failure, recovery will be strengthened. It is unrealistic to believe that every addict who commits to recovery will instantly live a perfect recovery life, and never give a thought to her previous addiction. Appropriately handling slips, or mistakes, can help one mature, grow, and move forward. These are a few suggestions for how to manage slips:

- Recognize that simply because one mistake has occurred, it doesn't have to be followed by many more.
- Don't give in to despair, thinking that because a slip has occurred, failure is unavoidable.
- Get immediate help and support. Have a list of supporters with their phone numbers handy and make a call for help without delay.
- Leave the area of the slip. Get to safer ground as soon as possible.

- If the slip happened at home, have a trustworthy person clear the area of any addictive material or paraphernalia before returning.
- Analyze the circumstances surrounding the slip. See what can be learned, so that preparations can be made to avoid the slip in the future.
- Consider ways to strengthen one's recovery. Go to more support meetings for awhile, read an inspirational book related to recovery, go to a weekend retreat designed for recovering addicts, or grow by giving to others.

 Fact

Women are less likely to relapse than men are. This is primarily due to the fact that women are more likely to seek treatment, engage in group counseling, and follow through with treatment recommendations. Hopefully, men will gain these same benefits as it becomes more socially acceptable for all individuals to seek and receive treatment.

It is critical for the recovering addict to recognize that when the slip is over, it's over. A recovering lifestyle begins again immediately. The second the beer bottle is put down, the cigarette is stomped out, the computer is turned off, recovery begins anew. It can begin with new insights, new awareness, and new appreciation for the hard work that recovery requires.

Be Aware of High-Risk Situations

High-risk situations have gone beyond the trigger point. These are situations in which relapse is imminent unless immediate steps are taken to protect one's recovery. You will recall that addictions are often a means of dealing with painful emotions, stress, and mental health problems. High-risk situations might be those instances in which painful emotions are on the surface. A wife announces she wants a divorce, a parent has been diagnosed with a terminal illness, one's best friend is killed in war, or a beloved child has been hit by a car. These are 911 situations, and for a recovering addict, the magnitude of these horrendous life circumstances may be overwhelming. As in any emergency situation, the recovering addict needs to call in all resources to help him cope with the tragedy and maintain recovery.

Alert

Chronic relapse occurs when the recovering addict repeatedly returns to his addictive behaviors and lifestyle. It is damaging and discouraging to both the addict and his family. Chronic relapse may be due to isolation from support, returning to living and social situations where addictive lifestyles are ongoing, or other stressful situations the recovering addict was not prepared to manage.

Life and death emergencies are not the only high-risk situations a recovering addict might encounter. There may be an exacerbation of mental or physical illness, such as a manic episode for someone with bipolar illness. A person with schizophrenia might experience a psychotic episode. Someone suffering from PTSD might be having a particularly difficult time with flashbacks. A cancer patient may discover another lump that is malignant and require further surgery. These situations may be strong pulls to self-medicate with the old addictions. The loss of a job, a car accident, or the trauma of weather disasters requiring costly repairs are further high-risk situations. Although these may seem like extreme circumstances that always happen to someone else, in truth, they are common life events that are displayed daily on the news. One cannot go through life and not experience these things oneself or see loved ones going through trying times.

The recovering addict cannot afford to manage this type of situation by relapsing and returning to his addiction. One must remember that the addiction didn't make life better before, and it won't make life better again.

Essential

> It is common to experience strong emotions such as anger, self-pity, resentment, bitterness, and grief when catastrophic life circumstances occur. Hanging on to these intense emotions is dangerous for the recovering addict. Get help! Contact a spiritual leader, a therapist, or a trusted friend or family member for help to work through these understandable, but potentially destructive, emotions.

Evaluating Relationships

There has already been a great deal of discussion about the importance of supportive relationships. Loyal friends who are understanding of the addict's struggles are invaluable for successful recovery. Unfortunately, not all friendships are positive or beneficial. The recovering addict will need to learn how to evaluate and cultivate the types of friendships that will support her recovery. Many addicts have histories of abuse and/or mental health problems that may make it difficult to accurately determine the motives and character of potential friends. When an addict makes the choice to attain freedom from his addiction, he's also choosing to take his life in unfamiliar and, often uncomfortable, directions.

An excellent friend is a welcome accompaniment. A significant problem that a recovering addict often encounters is what to do about friends with whom she shared her addictive lifestyle. The seemingly harsh response is, that if those friends are not willing to journey the path of recovery with the addict, the recovering addict will need to let them go. It is one more loss that may be quite painful, but it will be necessary in order to preserve recovery.

How does one evaluate friendships? These are some significant questions to ask oneself:

- Is he truthful?
- Does he say what he means, and mean what he says?
- Does he share the similar value of an addiction-free life?
- Can he tolerate and support the recovering addict's healthy life changes?
- Can he forgive a slip and firmly, but gently, support a return to recovery?
- Can he be trusted to keep sensitive information about the recovering addict's past confidential?
- Is he able to demonstrate empathy for the recovering addict without pity?
- Does he have a healthy sense of humor, joining with the recovering addict in having addiction-free fun?

Remember, it takes time to find and nurture solid, healthy friendships that will strengthen one's recovery and bring satisfying social fulfillment for a lifetime.

 Question

What is a sponsor?
A sponsor is someone involved in a twelve-step program who has time and experience in recovery. This person, as part of her own recovery, takes on the responsibility of mentoring a recovering addict newer in the program. A sponsor provides encouragement, support, and guidance in recovery and is a great resource to a recovering addict struggling with temptations to relapse.

Developing Healthy Self-Esteem

Developing healthy self-esteem is the best offensive action one can take to prevent relapse. Healthy self-esteem is often misperceived as always thinking positively of oneself and ignoring anything to the contrary. This definition is simply not accurate; in reality, it describes an attitude of arrogance and haughtiness. Healthy self-esteem is a well-rounded, honest, and accurate view of oneself. It involves taking a look at the whole picture.

 Fact

> Many recovering addicts struggle with feelings of inadequacy and low self-esteem. They may think of their lives as hopeless, worthless, and disastrous. The fact is that the addiction is the disaster, not the recovering addict. The alcohol, cocaine, gambling, pornography, food, and prescription drugs are the problems. Accurately identifying the problem (the addiction, not the addict), signals progress is ahead.

Each individual has gifts, talents, skills, abilities, assets, and creative interests. She also has problems, makes mistakes, commits wrongs, falls short, and has things to learn. The recovering addict may need to reconnect with the positives—she may be quite intelligent, artistic, funny, musical, articulate, and so forth. She may also have depression, anxiety, problems with stealing, and an addictive history of hurting others with lying and deceptions. Developing healthy self-esteem means that she will need to use her intelligence to plan for recovery, develop her talents as alternatives to engaging in her addiction, and allow her funny side to help her build positive relationships.

The recovering addict with healthy self-esteem will also need to get treatment for her mental health problems, pay back what she's stolen, apologize for lying to others, and commit to learning healthier behaviors. Honesty without excessive pride or self-denigration equals healthy self-esteem.

Keep the Support Going!

Simply because one is headed on the path toward solid recovery does not mean that support systems are no longer needed. In fact, they are needed as much as or more than ever. Over time, the memories of what it was like to be engulfed in a life of addictions might become dim. Memories of the addictive lifestyle might even take on a nostalgic or romantic glow. Support systems continue to hold one accountable, holding the recovering addict to a realistic perspective of where he's come from and reminding him of where he needs to go. Healthy support systems provide the recovering addict with friendships and activities that support his new, addiction-free life. Having one's social needs met without the trappings of addiction is one of the best ways to avoid relapse. As a person gains strength in recovery, he will also be able to provide more self-support. Taking initiative in making life changes such as moving to a new neighborhood, making new friends, and developing new interests is part of supporting one's own recovery. Sharing this with supportive friends makes recovery even sweeter!

 Alert

Self-pity is one of the biggest stumbling blocks for a recovering addict. One must resist the tendency to feel sorry for oneself. "Why me?" "Poor me!" "Why do I have to deal with these problems and others don't?" These thoughts are self-defeating. Overcoming a problem such as addiction can become an incredible strength and nothing to be sorry about.

CHAPTER 19

Real-Life
Considerations

LIFE GOES ON, with or without addictions, for both the addict and his family. Addictions disrupt the normal and essential flow of managing a household, a job, and family relationships. Although the addict is aware of these things, while she's engrossed in her addiction she may feel powerless to deal with these issues and simply let things slide. However, once in recovery, responsibilities need to be faced. This can be frightening for both the addict and her family. Recovery involves managing real life without the influence of addictions. It can be done!

Someone Has to Pay the Bills

Financial problems are often one of the biggest stressors a recovering addict and her family must face. During the time of active addiction, income may have dropped because of time spent away from the job engaging in the addiction, and debt likely accumulated to pay for the addiction and trying to keep the household afloat. Once the decision to enter recovery is made, treatment costs are incurred. Although this is necessary and appropriate, it's still an additional and significant expense.

Financial stressors can put great strain on family relationships. Rebuilding financial health and credibility is an essential part of recovery. It will require realigning one's financial priorities. With hard work and discipline, it can be accomplished.

What about Debt?

Recovery must come first! Without recovery, any financial progress will be temporary at best. The first step to dealing with debt is to get an accurate accounting of the financial picture. This will include how much money is owed to whom, and for what, as well as available assets. This may require help from others whose financial interests are tied to the recovering addict. Realize in advance that this process may be frustrating, anxiety-provoking, and discouraging. This is one of those times when the recovering addict needs a plan in place to prevent slips and/or relapse. The plan might include having a trusted friend or family member present to help, having a list of positive affirmations to read often, playing soothing music in the background, or saying a prayer before one begins. Take frequent breaks for relaxation and exercise. If the financial picture looks bleak, don't despair.

 Fact

It is important not to panic when one realizes that finances are in poor shape. Stay calm, get help, and develop a plan for financial recovery. Panic leads to decisions that typically make matters worse in the end. Above all, don't borrow more money or charge more on credit cards thinking this will be a quick fix to make ends meet. Be patient—an effective plan can be developed.

Focusing on financial losses, debt, and financial mistakes already made will not help. It will only make things worse. Instead, focus on realistic steps that can be taken to move forward. What are some of those steps? Consider these:

- **Take a financial planning seminar.** These are offered frequently in community adult education programs, at community colleges, or other community settings. Frequently, one can find these seminars for free or for minimal charge.

- **Consult with a financial planner to get expert, objective opinions on managing one's finances.** There are also many online financial planning resources, such as *http://financialplan .about.com* and *www.ameriprise.com*. It is also common for banks to offer free financial planning services if one has an account with them.
- **Get legal advice if necessary.** Bankruptcy should be a last resort and not considered as "an easy way out." In most situations, bankruptcy can be avoided. If this route is taken, consult an attorney to get an accurate perspective on what must be done, and the accurate consequences of these actions. There may be free legal aid services in your community if an attorney is unaffordable.
- **Consult a debt consolidation company.** These companies can help with negotiations with creditors and arrange payback plans. Not all of these companies are reputable. Do some homework before making a decision. Check with your local Better Business Bureau, your state attorney general, and consumer complaint websites to ensure that the company you select is a reputable one.
- **Create a detailed budget and stick to it.** A professional financial planner may be used, or there are many books and computer programs available that provide guidance with budget planning. If helpful, one's sponsor, trusted friend, or family member may be an accountability partner in this endeavor.
- **Cut up all credit cards.** Credit cards may seem like an easy fix when one is short of cash and resources. However, it is too easy to lose track of what is spent. Further debt can accumulate quickly and then one is worse off than ever. Additionally, credit card companies often charge exorbitant interest rates that also increase one's debt load.
- **Call one's creditors individually.** Many times creditors are more than willing to set up payment plans, or even forgo interest in order to recoup at least a portion of lost money.

- **Get a temporary second job to pay down debt.** This option is only viable if it doesn't threaten one's recovery.
- **Friends or family members may be able and willing to help financially.** However, for the sake of recovery, a payback plan should be developed and followed. An essential element of recovery is to take full responsibility for one's actions.
- **Charitable organizations, such as churches, often have funds available to offer emergency financial help.** Again, keeping recovery in mind, payback should be made when one is able, even if it isn't required.

Essential

If hiring a financial planner is not in your budget, there are some less expensive alternatives. Suze Orman is a well known financial advisor who has a number of books on the market as well as a website, *www.suzeorman.com*, where you can access information. Dave Ramsey's book, *The Total Money Makeover*, is filled with excellent financial advice, and he also has a website, *www.daveramsey.com*.

Taking these steps will go a long way to helping one regain financial health and recovery. Repaying debt and developing a financially responsible lifestyle also contribute greatly to one's self-esteem and self-worth.

What about My Job?

Having a job is a necessary part of life for most people. For the recovering addict, this may be another source of intense stress. There are many job-related issues a recovering addict may need to address. For example, he may have been fired, he may have worked with using coworkers, he may have developed a reputation for sloppy work, or he may have engendered animosity from coworkers who had to take on a greater workload. If a person has taken a leave of absence to get addiction treatment, he may have concerns about what to tell an employer or coworkers.

Again, before tackling job-related problems make sure that your recovery is protected by having a relapse protection plan in place. First, assess what your job situation was prior to your entering recovery. Important questions to consider include:

- What was the relationship like with your employer?
- What were relationships like with coworkers?
- Historically, what was the pattern of work evaluations?
- Was the job personally and financially satisfying?
- Was there anything related to the job situation that contributed to your addiction?
- Was the job well suited to your interests, abilities, and training?
- Was the work environment personally and emotionally safe?
- Were there opportunities for career advancement and increasing financial compensation?
- What was the company attitude toward employee addictions —supportive or punitive?

The answers to these questions will give you guidance and direction about what to do next. In considering how to approach your job situation during recovery, principles of twelve-step programs are helpful to remember. Some of those guiding principles include honesty with oneself and others, taking responsibility for one's actions, making amends where possible, and giving back. If returning to your job is a possibility and it appears this choice would work with recovery, have a meeting with your employer to get off on the right foot. Be honest with the employer about the disease of addiction, steps being taken to recover, and immediate goals related to work.

Listen carefully to one's employer about expectations for returning to work. This may mean drug testing, computer filters, a probation period, or extra supervision. Complying with these expectations in a positive manner is important in demonstrating that recovery is being taken seriously. It is important for the recovering addict to get to work on time, to have an excellent work ethic, and most of all, to display a positive attitude.

A recovering addict will need to consider carefully what to tell coworkers. If there are a few coworkers who are trustworthy, it will likely be helpful to take them into one's confidence and share one's struggle with addictions. They can provide much-needed support for the recovering addict returning to work. Besides, if no one knows the truth, imaginations can run wild. The resulting rumors generated may be far worse than the actual truth. This is not to say that any coworker needs to know all the details. Judge carefully how much to tell, but what one does tell must be the truth. Lying is associated with active addiction. Even though it might seem that lying will make things easier when returning to work, in reality, it's a setup for relapse. A supportive employer, your sponsor, and your therapist may be very helpful in thinking this through.

 Alert

It is in an employer's best interest to support your recovery. Employers are quite aware of the costs of addiction and treatment to the company. Therefore, many employers allow and encourage twelve-step meetings on the job site where recovering employees may gain help and support either during breaks or after work hours. Take advantage if this is available.

Some employers and coworkers may not provide the support that you would desire. In fact, they might respond with criticism, putdowns, and unfair expectations. A recovering addict will need to prepare with the "what if" exercise so as not to be taken off guard should these unfortunate events occur. Some coworkers, or even bosses, may have been "using buddies" and resent a change in the relationship. They might even feel threatened by another's recovery, reminded of their own problems with addiction. Do not allow these negative reactions to sabotage recovery! Call in all support systems to help. Hopefully, with perseverance, sensitivity, and understanding, others will make positive changes as well and the work situation will improve. If not, it may very well be time to look for other employment. This could even be an opportunity to consider a new career.

Who's Going to Take Out the Trash?

The day-to-day life of a recovering addict is going to look very different from his "using" days. It will look different for his family also. In the beginning, neither the recovering addict nor his family may know what to expect. There may also be lingering resentments and blame held by family members who had to pick up the slack prior to recovery.

 Fact

Taking on excessive commitments at home, or at work, out of guilt because of irresponsible behavior while engaging in one's addiction is counterproductive. One should also beware of trying to pay back family members with gifts, promises, or taking over their chores. If possible, part-time responsibilities are appropriate as recovery is being established. Balance is the key.

Even after recovery begins, the addict may be so focused on the process of recovery (attending support groups, outpatient therapy, and so forth) that family members may feel that nothing has changed in terms of household responsibilities. A time for clearing the air is in order. Depending on the severity of the situation, family therapy may be helpful in working through painful feelings. The recovering addict will need to take responsibility for not being present, physically or emotionally, to take out the trash, repair the dishwasher, and help with laundry. A parent will need to own up to the fact that he didn't take time to help children with their homework. Family members will need an opportunity to respectfully express feelings they've held toward the addict around these issues.

Family members also need to take responsibility for behaving disrespectfully toward the addict, for purposely hurting her to get even for their own pain, and for not taking care of themselves emotionally. These are only examples of the dynamics that will likely need to be worked through before a realignment of household responsibilities can take place successfully. At this point, a family meeting will be helpful to discuss with one another each member's responsibility for managing the household. Expectations need to be clear and understanding affirmed.

 Alert

Lying and unkept promises may be used to try and smooth over difficult family situations and painful emotions. These are old and familiar coping mechanisms for the addict, and therefore comfortable to slip back on. However, for the addict in recovery, these tactics won't work.

While the recovering addict may fully desire the establishment of a healthy household, he may also have feelings of fear and ambivalence. He may fear that he won't measure up, that he'll fail, or that he'll relapse and spoil everything once again. The ambivalence is that, in spite of his fears, he wants more than anything to move forward with recovery. And recovery means taking responsibility. Initially, the recovering addict will need to be honest about what he's able to do around the house. Solid recovery is still the primary objective for the recovering addict. He may have therapy sessions to attend, twelve-step support meetings to attend, medical appointments to keep, legal issues to attend to, and/or community service to perform. There may also be a learning curve to consider as the recovering addict is learning how to do household skills never before attempted. Patience, understanding, and kindness will be necessary for everyone to get through this phase of change.

Maintaining Healthy Relationships

A recovering addict, who has spent most of her past time with "using" friends, or at least friends sympathetic to addictions, may feel uncertainty about what defines a healthy relationship. For someone new in recovery, caution is in order.

Essential

Learn to have fun without addictions. This may be a challenge, but it's an excellent way to begin cementing healthy relationships. Games without gambling, healthy foods, and soda rather than alcohol really can be enjoyable. There may be old friends that were bypassed when addictions took over that would be willing to reconnect over healthy fun. Invite them over!

When drastically changing one's course in life, it is a temptation to want to lean on others. It may still be difficult to know whom to trust. Someone who appears extremely nice, helpful, and compassionate may be exactly that, or he might be co-dependent and interfere with the difficult work recovery will take. Romantic relationships, in particular, should be avoided when one is new in recovery. The emotional highs of new romance may even feel comparable to the high of addictions. One's judgment about relationships may not be trustworthy in this state. Even new friendships can take a lot of time and energy to develop and may detract from recovery efforts. The mantra for a newly recovering addict is wait, be patient, and work toward a healthy, solid recovery. Only when a person is healthy herself will she be ready to recognize and participate in new, healthy relationships. Someone who has been heavily involved in an addictive lifestyle for a long time may not feel comfortable with her own identity, much less learning that of a new person. However, the desire to leave the old, addictive lifestyle and the insecurities that may exist in moving forward can leave a person quite vulnerable. Any friendly person might appear to be just what is needed.

Fresh recovery is often a time of loneliness. A person has left behind "using" friends, but may not have yet developed healthy friends. This interim period is fragile and needs to be handled as such. It should be used to strengthen recovery efforts, to evaluate personal goals, and to find peace within oneself.

 Question

What about dating someone in the support group?
Although this sounds like a good idea since that person understands what it's like to struggle with addictions, in reality, it is unlikely to support recovery for either party. Problems due to an overly dependent relationship, a shift in focus from recovery to the other person, and replacing the euphoria of addiction with the euphoria of a new relationship all spell danger for healthy recovery.

Effective Time Management

More than likely, when actively involved in addiction, a good chunk of your time was spent fantasizing about the addiction, planning how to get time for the addiction, figuring out how to get money for the addiction, actually engaging in the addiction, recuperating from the addiction, and hiding the addiction from others. Often even eating and sleeping may have been sacrificed to get all that done. Once in recovery, time that was spent on addictions needs to be filled with healthy activities. A person may feel overwhelmed with how to fill the now empty spaces. However, time vacancies or time used unproductively may be triggers for slips and/or relapses. Successful recovery will require learning how to use one's time in a way that produces healthy growth.

The good news is that effective time management is a skill that can be learned. Here are some tips:

- Get organized. Purchasing a day planner, a calendar, and other necessary supplies for planning and keeping track of important dates is a start.
- Prioritize tasks and activities. Initially, brainstorming every-thing one can think of that must be done gets things out on the table. Then, go through the list and prioritize the items from most to least important.
- Based on the identified priorities, set personal goals. There should be both short-term and long-term goals. Goals are essential for keeping a person focused on the future rather than dwelling on the past.
- Make a "to do" list each day, either before one goes to bed in preparation for the next day or first thing in the morning. Pri-oritize the "to do" list.
- If there are any tasks on your "to do" list that seem overwhelm-ing, break them down into smaller, more manageable chunks.
- Regularly evaluate how the time management plan is work-ing. Especially at first, this should be done on a weekly basis. Make adjustments if necessary to ensure success.

These suggestions will guarantee that the most important things in one's life get done first. Following these guidelines will also provide forward momentum that will increasingly build self-confidence and self-esteem. Remember that recovery must be at the top of the list!

Avoid Pitfalls

There are pitfalls that a person must avoid in order to succeed with effective time management. Perfectionism and lack of flexibility are prime culprits. Plans, lists, and goals are all guidelines. They provide a framework and structure to keep a person on track. No one can accurately predict the future. Life's unexpected twists and turns require flexibility to navigate. Perfection will certainly never be reached in one's lifetime. Look for growth and forward progress to measure addiction recovery. Striving for perfection will only lead to feelings of failure and frustration.

Another pitfall is the excessive desire to please others. While it's nice to see others enjoy one's gifts and efforts, taking care of one's recovery first will be the best gift of all. What this means is that the recovering addict will need to learn how to say NO loud and clear when necessary. A recovering addict may have to redefine his personal boundaries. This will also mean he has to communicate what those boundaries are to others. Respectfully saying no is a skill to be learned in establishing healthy boundaries.

 Fact

Executive coaches, mentors, personal or career coaches are all people who may be of great help with getting time management back on track. These are individuals with varying levels of professional training. Their objective is to help a person become confident, organized, and goal directed. Check out credentials, references, and training before engaging their services.

Finally, procrastination is probably the biggest roadblock of all when it comes to preventing effective time management. The reasons why someone procrastinates will need exploration in order to break through and move forward.

Some of the causes of procrastination are:

- **Difficult and unpleasant tasks.** Do these first and get them out of the way. This will eliminate the sense of dread that exists when they're left for later.
- **Work that seems overwhelming.** Huge workloads or work that seems overwhelming because it requires new learning and is unfamiliar needs to be broken down into bite-size morsels.
- **Vague goals that are not clearly defined.** Spending time clarifying one's goals will save time in the long run.
- **Overcommitting.** This may occur out of a desire to please others. Learn to commit to only those things that can be realistically accomplished.
- **Waiting until the last minute.** This may be a habit that develops from the other reasons for procrastination. Sometimes a person will mistakenly believe he can't get anything done without the adrenaline rush of last-minute pressure. This may be related to old addictive behaviors and needs to change.
- **Fear of failure.** A person may believe that it's better not to try at all rather than to try and fail. This is NOT true. Trying itself is something to value.
- **Fear of change.** This fear is based on the belief that change will be bad, difficult, and have disastrous consequences. Change will occur whether one wants it or not. It is far better to work on creating a change that is most likely to promote recovery.

 Question

Can someone become addicted to procrastination?
The adrenaline rush of waiting until the last minute to complete an assignment, waiting until the pressure is insurmountable, may resemble that of addiction. The recovering addict must ask herself if this could be a trigger or a substitute for the euphoria of addiction. If so, she should be honest and deal with the problem in recovery work.

Many of the causes of procrastination have fear at the root. These fears must be faced and seen for what they really are. Many times fears are based on assumptions and distortions, not reality. Effective time management will give the recovering addict the skill and confidence to take care of her "recovering business."

You Can Be a Good Parent and Help Yourself

The reality is that helping yourself is being a good parent. Children need to see good self-care modeled. In reconnecting with one's children, honesty regarding one's addiction is essential. Of course, this honesty will need to be appropriate for the child's age and developmental level. In being honest with them about addictions, you need to let your children know that, for a while anyway, recovery needs to come first. This is not to say that the recovering addict should not give children time and attention. The important thing is not to make promises and also not to make demands. Children will likely remember too many broken promises and will be resentful of demands.

 Fact

Resiliency is the ability to recover from adversity, trauma, or difficult life circumstances. Children are often quite resilient. They want a healthy parent committed to recovery. Fear that one's children will never forgive the mistakes made during active addiction should not be allowed to sabotage recovery.

Key elements of good parenting when one is new in recovery are:

- Honesty at the child's level.
- Follow-through. Don't say that something will happen or get done unless there is complete certainty that follow-through is a surety.

- At the child's level, allow him to see his parent engaging in activities to improve and grow.
- Treat the child with respect.
- Make certain the child knows that her parent's addiction is not her fault.
- Allow the child to express his painful emotions.
- Reconnect with one's child slowly, at a pace comfortable and doable for the recovering addict, and at the same time, being sensitive to the child's lack of trust and faith in his formerly addictive parent.
- If age appropriate, encourage one's child to participate in family therapy and/or in support groups.
- Allow the child to ask questions about what is going on in her family.

Being a good parent does not mean being a perfect parent. It means doing the best one can, giving liberal amounts of sincere apology when necessary, and continuing to learn ways of doing it better. A good parent reassures the child that he is loved and wanted, no matter what, and in spite of both the parent's and the child's imperfections.

Restoring Credibility in the Community

Restoring one's credibility in the community will take time and patience. People in the recovering addict's community will want to see evidence that the changes are genuine and lasting. The only way this will happen is to consistently live a recovery lifestyle.

For the recovering addict, the first step in restoring public credibility is to work through any feelings of personal shame or embarrassment at having had an addiction. Although many in the community will be supportive, there will also be those who will not. Again, it is helpful to have a plan in advance as to how to deal with these unpleasant encounters. In the beginning, the best method is to quietly go about the business of recovery. Restoring trust and respect through the modeling of a changed life is the one tried and true means of regaining credibility. Performing community service as a consequence of one's addiction may be required. If so, do it well and with a positive attitude. Lies and deception may have built a reputation of being dishonest for the addict. As a recovering addict, honesty is *always* the best policy and the only way to turn the tide. Once a recovering addict is feeling more secure with his recovery, giving back to the community will demonstrate sincerity that things are different. It will also help the recovering addict to grow in self-respect.

 Alert

Even though supportive people may graciously tell the recovering addict that he doesn't have to repay a debt, apologize for a wrong done to others, and so on, restoring credibility requires making amends. Making amends is a cornerstone of twelve-step programs for good reason. They can be a public demonstration that the recovering addict means business.

One may give back by helping other addicts in their recovery process. Work in educating the public on the dangers of addiction. If the recovering addict feels comfortable, being transparent about her own journey may help encourage others. Helping with community beautification projects, serving in one's place of worship, or volunteering to help in times of community crisis are only a few examples of how one can give back. One might even seek public office, serve on the city council, or lobby to change laws related to addiction. A consistent life of honesty, integrity, and hard work is difficult to criticize. Credibility can be re-established, but it will take time.

CHAPTER 20

How Addictions Affect Family Members

ADDICTIONS CAN AFFECT every facet of life for the addict and his family. To deny this is not only to minimize the problem, but also to minimize one's level of recovery. It is common for family members to go through stages of denial, self-deception, anger, and fear as they grieve over the cost of addictions for someone they love. Often family members feel lost, wanting desperately to help, but are unsure what to do or where to start. Families, as well as addicts, need to learn how to recover.

Damaged Family Bonds

Addictions change the dynamics in a family system. Trust is broken, feelings of safety may be in jeopardy, and uncertainty about the future looms over everyone's head. Initially, family members may have been misled by lies and deceptions, unable to believe that their loved one could have changed so much. Addictions change a person's moods and thinking processes. Once addictions take hold, the addict's priorities change as well. The addiction takes priority over relationships. The loving, honest individual that family members knew may be hidden behind the screen of addictions.

Based on warm memories, family members may become enablers in their attempts to help the addict return to the person they remembered. Enabling is anything a person does that makes it easier for the addict to obtain and use his substance or engage in his compulsive behaviors. Here are some examples of enabling:

- Paying the addict's debts
- Making excuses for the addict's behaviors
- Lying to the addict's boss when she doesn't want to go to work because of a hangover
- Continuing to forgive addictive behaviors that are inexcusable
- Ignoring suspicious addictive behaviors as if they never happened
- Refusing to hold an addict accountable for rude, abusive behaviors
- Taking over household responsibilities that the addict should rightfully be sharing

Frequently, family members blame themselves for their loved one becoming involved in addictions. Enabling can be a way of trying to soothe one's conscience. It is also a way of trying to draw the addict back into family relationships. Although family members believe they are trying to help with enabling behaviors, the opposite is true.

 Fact

Recovery requires accountability. Initially, the addict may resent accountability, believing it restricts her personal freedom. Family members may resist holding the addict accountable out of fear the addict will rebel and the situation will worsen. The fact is that accountability releases family members from their fears and frees the addict to pursue recovery and a healthy future.

Enabling prolongs denial on all parts and allows the addict to avoid facing his disease of addiction. This means that treatment and recovery are postponed, allowing the addiction to progress to a more serious, and perhaps, more lethal stage. When enabling doesn't work, family members may change tactics and try to control the addict.

Telling the addict what he has to do, where he can go, and with whom he can associate typically leads to angry shouting matches. The intent to redirect the addict away from his addiction is good, but ineffective. When it seems that every attempt to help their addicted loved one has failed, family members may withdraw in despair. At this point, family members may try to continue their own lives as usual, hiding painful emotions as they watch their loved one deteriorate. Relationships are damaged and it may feel that the addiction has gained the upper hand. It doesn't have to stay this way.

Dealing with Difficult Emotions

Confusion, fear, disappointment, anger, and hurt only begin to describe the myriad of painful emotions that family members feel when a loved one becomes involved in addictions. These feelings are legitimate and common in this situation.

Painful emotions associated with addictions can imprison a family. If not addressed, these painful emotions can lead to family members developing hatred for their family system. Apathy and indifference may result as ways to escape. This doesn't have to happen. With help, family members can work through painful emotions.

When painful emotions seem to dominate one's life, it's time to take action. Family members also need support, encouragement, and, many times, professional help. Recovery is not only the desired result for the addict, but also for families. Once family members recognize their own need for recovery, the process may begin. In dealing with difficult emotions, family members must be able to separate their own emotions from those of the addict. As hard as it may be to accept, family members have no power to control what the addict feels or what she does. This brings up the idea of sympathy versus empathy. Sympathy is feeling sorry for someone. It carries the implication that "we'll all sink together." While this may provide companionship in one's misery, it's not helpful. Empathy is imagining oneself in another person's situation as much as possible, recognizing the problem, offering to help, but refusing to become part of the problem just so the one in trouble doesn't feel alone. An empathic person maintains his own well-being, staying on emotional solid ground, while at the same time offering support and practical help to the one suffering.

Family members of addicts must become empathic, avoiding the pitfalls of being sympathetic. This will require strengthening their own emotional, psychological, and physical health. From this position of strength, they are better able to help their loved one when she's ready to enter recovery.

Alert

> Overly sympathetic family members inhibit the addict's recovery rather than help it. Sympathy gives the addict permission to feel sorry for himself. It implies that recovery is just too hard and unattainable. This is not true. Family members need to let the addict know that, although recovery is hard, it is possible, and they are there to help.

So how do family members enter recovery? First, acknowledge the painful emotions. They're real, they're justified, and they have a purpose. Ignoring them, hiding them, excusing them, and pretending they don't exist only make painful emotions worse. It doesn't make them go away. Do not be ashamed or embarrassed about painful emotions. Get help to deal with them if necessary.

Professional counselors and/or spiritual leaders are trained to help people with difficult emotions. Support groups, such as Al-Anon, provide opportunities to hear that others in similar situations are experiencing the same problems. It can be a relief to realize that one is not alone or strange. This is also a time for self-examination. Recall that addictions and mental health disorders often have a genetic component. Family members may need to face troubling behaviors and moods themselves. Consult with a medical professional to see if medications might be helpful.

Remember the old adage "misery loves company." It's true. When an addict is in the midst of her addiction, the tendency is for her to want to share the misery. Family members need to learn not to accept that misery as their own. Again, this is where boundaries come into play. Emotional boundaries are just as important to establish as physical boundaries. If an addict is angry or depressed in relation to his addiction, family members do not also have to feel angry or depressed. The feelings of the addict need to be *his* feelings. They do not need to be treated as a virus, an infection to be spread around to anyone in the vicinity. When the addict is ready for recovery, he will have to deal with his own difficult emotions. Once family members have acknowledged, faced, and dealt with the understandable painful emotions they have, they are in a position to move forward in their recovery. They are also in a more solid position to help their loved one in recovery.

 Question

What are emotional boundaries?
Emotional boundaries, like physical boundaries, involve limits. Emotional boundaries do not keep one's emotions trapped within, but rather, allow for the honest expression of one's emotions and the prevention of the emotions of others from encroaching. Family members do not have to take on the addict's emotions of anger, depression, and discouragement as if they were their own.

Communication Is Key

Opening the doors to communication is an important first step in reestablishing healthy family relationships. Basically, real communication is being able to give and receive accurate messages.

Accuracy is the key, as people often communicate through the filters of their own perceptions and beliefs that may not be shared by others. This leads to distorted messages that build into misunderstandings. Listening is the foundation to effective communication. Genuine listening focuses on understanding and learning from the other person involved in the conversation. Often one listens out of a desire to self-protect. "Am I in danger of getting hurt?" "Am I in danger of someone taking advantage of me?" "Am I in danger of being attacked?" These are all common questions one asks when listening with the motive of self-protection. When interacting with an addict whose behaviors have been hurtful and frightening, this is understandable. However, in order for the situation to improve, the goals of listening must change. The focus must be on understanding the message of the speaker, not on self-protection. This task is much easier when appropriate emotional boundaries have been put in place. Genuine listening does not mean that one will agree with everything heard; it just means that one will accurately hear the message.

 Fact

Body language is equally as important as the language of words. Posture, facial expressions, hand gestures, and body position all communicate messages in powerful ways. Effective communication takes body language into consideration. A defensive posture can quickly negate encouraging words. A person needs to be just as aware of what she's saying with her body as she is with her words.

Questions asking for clarification or further information will often be necessary to get a complete, accurate message. Repeating back what one thinks he's heard and asking the speaker if he's heard correctly is another method to promote effective communication. These questions also reassure the speaker that there is a real desire to understand and a heartfelt caring in the communication. Two words to avoid in effective communication are "You" and "Why." These two words imply attacks and accusations. The typical reaction of the hearer is to respond with defensiveness.

The focus of the communication then shifts from understanding to winning—who is going to come out on top, the winner. The speaker will have better communication results when beginning sentences with "I." This implies taking personal responsibility, allowing the hearer space to have her own thoughts and opinions. These communication skills may not have been the pattern in families dealing with an addicted loved one. Frequently there will have been so much hurt, pain, and anger in communications that a defensive position has seemed the only safe approach. Therefore, it will take time and practice to change the communication environment to one of safety, allowing for concern, thoughts, and feelings to be expressed without fear.

Essential

> Assertive communication is a style of communicating in which someone speaks directly regarding what he feels, thinks, and desires. An assertive person asks for what he wants, but not at the expense of the rights and feelings of others. The goal of assertive communication is to maintain self-respect, while at the same time doing everything possible to enhance relationships.

Constructive Fighting

Conflict is inevitable in relationships where addiction is a third party. The lies, blame, accusations, and fears that often accompany addictions make conflict unavoidable.

Conflict has the potential to deeply damage family relationships. One might ask if it's even possible to fight constructively. Absolutely! However, constructive fighting does involve learning some new communication skills, following some basic ground rules, and above all, respecting one's opponent. Again, this doesn't mean agreeing with another, but respecting each other's basic rights to have thoughts, feelings, and opinions of your own.

Constructive conflict is a process. Many feel that in the heat of conflict, it's impossible to be thoughtful about process. If one is too angry or upset to engage in the process, it's better to take some time alone to cool down before entering into conflict resolution. The following steps describe the process of constructive conflict:

- Take a few seconds to decide if addressing this conflict is worthwhile. Is the upsetting issue a petty irritation that can be attributed to a bad day at work, or is it significant to the well-being of the relationship?
- Choose a time for the conflict when there are no distractions and there will be adequate time to process the conflict.
- The upset individual first states the facts from her perspective.
- She next states her feelings related to this matter. It is important to state the facts first, as feelings often make it difficult to be objective.
- She then states how she would like things to be different, what changes she would like to see take place.
- She next states what she will need to do if these changes don't take place. This is not a threat or manipulation, but merely a statement of her next move.
- Following these steps, the listener gets a turn. He responds with his own sense of the facts about the situation and states his feelings.
- Once facts and feelings are out in the open, discussion can occur where questions may be asked and clarification established.

Hopefully, the conclusion of the conflict will end in a satisfactory resolution for both parties. Other possibilities include compromising, taking time to gather additional information and postponing the conflict until better prepared, or agreeing to disagree.

Constructive conflict is predicated on some essential ground rules. Respect is the key. This means no derogatory name-calling, no condescending attitudes, no dismissing the other's point of view, and no intimidating tactics. It also means that if one person is becoming too angry or upset during the conflict, a call for time-out is respected. Other ground rules involve not bringing up past conflicts, staying focused on the issue at hand, and not intentionally saying hurtful things to the other person. This process may seem very mechanical at first, but as with any new skill, it will become easier and more natural with use and practice. When first learning the process of constructive conflict, start with small disagreements where the outcome will not have a serious impact on the relationship. For example, what meal to have for dinner or which car to drive to the park is, hopefully, not too emotionally laden for practice. For deeply wounded families who have engaged in destructive conflict for too long, professional counseling may be helpful.

Alert

> Accusations, negative labels, and demands are hallmarks of destructive fighting. They tend to shut down communication and further damage relationships rather than lead to conflict resolution. Empathy, understanding, and objective feedback are much more effective tools in resolving conflict. Communication that is other-centered instead of self-centered is more likely to achieve the goal of enhanced relationship.

A professional counselor is trained to teach communication techniques and can act as a coach while a family is learning to change their style of dealing with conflict. Constructive conflict does work and, when carried out effectively, can provide a family with a sense of satisfaction and accomplishment.

When Roles Are Reversed

Roles within the family often become reversed when one or more members are dealing with addictions. Parents may abdicate their role as provider/caretaker in favor of pursuing their addiction. Children then take over the role of parents, making certain the food is prepared, the laundry is done, and the bills are paid. Adult children who have previously been responsible may regress into childish behaviors once addictions take over. A boss who succumbs to addictions may allow subordinates to manage her business. An addicted spouse may leave the responsibilities of parenting, financial provision, and household management completely on the shoulders of the nonaddicted spouse. When roles are reversed, resentments can develop in family members. Family members may feel helpless to change the situation. They have likely made many requests to the addict to change, to pick up his share of the load, and to recognize the hardship he's placing on others in the family. As long as the addiction is in charge, these requests typically fall on deaf ears, so to speak.

Essential

Family members may have been dissatisfied with their roles in the first place. Before challenging the addict regarding role reversals, it might be helpful for family members to reflect on whether they were satisfied with previous roles. Personal therapy may be beneficial in exploring this issue. Being clear about what one wants will help one to ask with greater confidence.

Family members may take on a reactive stance, doing the addict's share of the work, but feeling angry and resentful. It is essential for recovery that family members become proactive in these situations. Here are some tips for how to manage situations of role reversal:

- Do not suppress feelings, but express them respectfully.
- Firmly, but respectfully, point out addictive behaviors that are unacceptable.

- Make clear requests designed to re-establish healthy family roles.
- If changes do not occur, or if requests are ignored, be prepared to warn the addict of impending consequences.
- If a warning of consequences also meets with a lack of cooperation, then the consequences must take place without fail and in a timely manner. Therefore, it is essential that family members don't threaten consequences that they are not willing or prepared to put into place.

Family members are often reluctant to enact these changes, fearing the addict will be driven further into her world of addictions or, even worse, will do something in response to the demands that will threaten her very life. Although an addiction is a disease, addictions do not make it impossible for the addict to make choices. Yes, it is more difficult for an addict to make a responsible choice than for others; however, it is still not impossible. An addict is not responsible for her disease, but she is responsible for her choices.

 Alert

Manipulation is a hallmark strategy of an addict. An addict may become very convincing in manipulating others to help him continue in his addiction. Family members must be aware of this tactic and not be taken in. If family members feel confused or uncertain, they need to check things out. Ask the addict direct questions, hold her accountable, and examine the evidence to verify the addict's assertions. Remember, straightforward honesty is the path to recovery.

Family members cannot force choices on the addict. Consequences may be what are necessary for the addict to recognize how deeply he has been negatively affected by the addictions. They may be the motivation an addict needs to enter recovery. At the very least, they are necessary for the family to enter recovery. A significant problem is when role reversals affect children, who are not capable or powerful enough to state expectations and carry out consequences. In this situation, extended family, adult friends, neighbors, teachers, or health care providers may need to report the situation to social services in order to make sure the children are cared for and protected.

The Effects of Financial Hardships

There is no question that addictions are expensive. They cost the addict, but quite often, family members are placed in financial hardship as well. Family members incur financial costs through theft, hiring additional help when the addict is functionally absent, paying for legal assistance, and paying for treatment. There are also financial hardships when the addict loses his job, spends money on his addictive substances or behaviors, or gambles away his paycheck. None of these are minor expenses, and family members may legitimately fear complete financial ruin as a result of addictions. Credit may be destroyed, and with that, the financial reputation of family members as well as the addict.

Financial hardship may be a source of shame and embarrassment for family members. Again, anger and resentment directed toward the addict are commonplace and understandable. Family members must be proactive in protecting themselves financially. It may be necessary to remove the addict's name from bank accounts, credit cards, and assets. This should not be seen as rejection of the addict, but recognition of the reality that when addictions are in charge, the addict is not the responsible individual that he may have been in the past. Family members have a right to protect themselves financially. Financial consequences need to land where they belong, with the addict. If family members choose to help the addict pay for treatment and recovery efforts, they have a right to choose resources they can afford. The most expensive, exclusive treatment programs will be worthless if the addict is not committed to recovery. If an addict is committed to recovery, even less-expensive treatment options will be of great benefit provided the professionals involved are adequately trained in working with addictions.

It is also important for family members to understand that requiring the addict to repay them financially is reasonable and necessary for the addict's recovery. It helps build the addict's self-esteem and helps heal the resentments family members may have experienced when financially struggling.

 Fact

> Making amends is a key component of twelve-step programs in working toward recovery. And for good reason. Making amends builds one's self-esteem, helps rebuild relationships, and makes it clear to others that one is serious about recovery. For family members to tell the addict that amends aren't necessary or required is to block his recovery progress.

Rebuilding Trust

The basis of trustworthiness is saying what one means, and meaning what one says. Trust is established when follow-through with one's promises happens in a timely and excellent manner. Trust can only flourish in the absence of lies and deceptions. Almost all of these conditions for trust are likely demolished when addictions take over one's life. Family members who are trying to rebuild trust with a recovering addict are not starting from scratch, but are trying to climb out of a deep well of hurt, disappointment, and fear. Rebuilding trust involves commitments from family members as well as the addict. Family members must commit to being honest with their feelings and their expectations. They must be clear on boundaries. The addict must commit to honesty and truthfulness regardless of the fallout. He must not only remain sober from his addictions, but also begin to make amends to people he's hurt with his addictions.

Family members and the addict must all be committed to taking down the defensive shields that were a hallmark of interaction during the height of the addiction. If slips or relapses occur, the addict must be honest with family members and allow them to see her steps to return to recovery. Start small. In rebuilding trust, it's better to make a small promise or commitment and keep it, rather than to make large promises that are impossible to manage. Genuinely focusing on the needs of others, paying attention to their feelings, and spending time and energy on building them up goes a long way in rebuilding trust.

Essential

The fear of being hurt again must be dealt with if trust is to be re-established. One must be realistic, but not fearful. Whether an addict or not, future mistakes are inevitable. However, future mistakes cannot be handled now. Avoiding trust because of fear of future hurts will prevent healing in relationships.

Establishing New and Healthy Family Relationships

Family recovery is possible; it can be rewarding, and relationships have the potential to be more meaningful than ever. In recovery, there may develop an honesty and openness that was never even dreamed of before. Family members in recovery will need to develop a vision of what makes up a healthy family. It is not uncommon that addictions run in families and may have affected families for generations. Thus, families may have little idea of what healthy interactions look like.

Taking the time to develop a vision for healthy family relationships is time well spent. Having no direction or idea of what one is working toward means a lot of unnecessary trial-and-error approaches. It can be frustrating and discouraging. Don't allow fear, pride, or shame to keep you from learning.

It's never too late to learn. Read books on healthy relationships, attend relationship workshops or seminars, watch respected role models to see how they interact, and/or ask for help from professional counselors. Once it becomes clear what healthy family relationships involve, goals and objectives can be set. It will take time, often more time than one would like, and perseverance. Celebrating every victory, every step taken forward, will make the process rewarding and worthwhile.

CHAPTER 21

Hope for a Balanced Life

THE NATURE OF addictions is to upset the balance in one's life. The dopamine pleasure circuit takes over the driver's seat, leading the addict down a pathway to sickness and trouble. Recovery is all about recovering a healthy balance, enabling the recovering addict and her family to enjoy all aspects of life. It may be that the recovering addict never knew a balanced life prior to her addictions. The process of learning and discovering what that means can be a joyful and rewarding experience.

The Mind-Body-Spirit Connection

Human beings are magnificently made. They are also creatures of great complexity. All aspects of one's humanity working in synchrony leads to balance. What a person thinks and feels emotionally can affect his physical and spiritual conditions. How he feels physically can affect thoughts, feelings, and spirituality. And spiritual health can help one rise above problems of the mind and body. Recovery is an excellent opportunity to take a personal inventory. Self-reflection is the first step in this process. An addict often loses the ability to self-evaluate and may ignore internal clues as to her state of health. Self-reflection is the beginning of training herself to accurately discern her state of being.

Additionally, it may be wise to get professional opinions as to one's state of health. A thorough physical examination will be important to determine if there are any residual effects from addictions.

If so, one's physician can make recommendations to further aid in physical recovery. Individual psychotherapy and a psychological evaluation, if indicated, can determine if there is any cognitive damage from addictions or lingering emotional problems. Consultation with a spiritual director or spiritual leader can help one evaluate spiritual health. Even though it is important to learn to trust one's own perceptions and instincts, objective input from neutral professionals can help point out things one may have missed. Armed with information from all angles, one is ready to proceed to a balanced recovery.

 ## Question

Once in recovery, will physical symptoms related to addictions go away?
It depends. With good health care, sobriety, and time, many of the physical symptoms brought on by addictions will resolve or, at the least, improve. For example, liver damage due to alcoholism is often reversible with sobriety. If symptoms persist after a significant time in recovery, a physician should be consulted.

Good Self-Care

Recovery must take priority in an addict's life. Although it may seem selfish to others, and even to the addict, it is really the most selfless thing an addict can do. Selfishness is continuing in one's addiction, further damaging oneself, others, and relationships. Good self-care begins with following the recommendations made by knowledgeable professionals after a thorough evaluation. Developing a follow-through plan will be helpful and will provide guidelines that make compliance easier.

For an addict, good self-care is a twofold process. The first component is protecting one's recovery. This means being aware of cravings and triggers that could provoke a slip or relapse. To pretend they will never occur again is to potentially set oneself up for problems and place one's recovery at risk. Triggers have already been addressed, but how does one manage cravings? Here are some suggestions:

- Don't deny the presence of cravings. Do wait them out. Most cravings will diminish or go away after about fifteen to twenty minutes.
- Change old patterns. Avoid places, people, and situations that may initiate cravings.
- Periodically remind oneself of the pain, unpleasantness, and negative consequences of addictions. This will give one strength to say no to cravings.
- Be patient. Cravings will get weaker and easier to manage with time in recovery.
- Have substitutes available. Chewing sugarless gum, eating healthy snacks, or engaging in a hobby that keeps one's hands busy are examples of substitutes.
- Keep the long-term goal of a balanced, healthy lifestyle constantly in sight.

The second component of good self-care is developing healthy habits that may or may not have been present prior to one's addiction. The development of healthy habits takes time. Allow at least a month for a new habit to take root. This is a time of testing and will require perseverance. After a month, one's new habit will become easier and a more natural part of one's daily life. Be patient. Healthy habits will pay big benefits over the span of one's life.

Remember, develop health habits that encompass balance. As part of one's overall plan for health, choose goals that address mental, physical, and spiritual health. For starters, reinforce healthy habits that may have been in place prior to one's addiction but were forgotten, neglected, or ignored. Once this is accomplished, add new habits one at a time. Habits related to physical health will include reaching and/or maintaining a healthy weight, eating healthy foods that won't trigger cravings, and exercise. Physical health is also about getting regular checkups such as recommended mammograms, stress tests, blood-sugar testing, colonoscopies, and so forth. Healthy eating in particular is essential for one's physical recovery. Addictions often deplete one's nutrients through malnutrition. Additionally, sugar and refined carbohydrates may trigger cravings for drugs and alcohol. Remember that alcohol is broken down into sugar during the digestive process and sugar itself can activate the dopamine pleasure circuit. Nutritional supplements may be necessary to regain physical balance. It may be wise to consult one's physician or a nutritionist trained in addiction recovery for nutritional guidelines.

 Alert

Alcohol can interfere with the absorption of calcium by the bones. Brittle bones may result, putting one at risk for bone fractures. As part of recovery, it will be important to get adequate calcium along with vitamin D, which helps metabolize calcium. One can get vitamin D from the sun or through fortified milk.

Physical health and development has many benefits. It provides one with the stamina to enjoy many other activities, promotes healthy weight management, and can prolong one's life. If exercise has not previously been a habit, take it slowly. Get physician approval before starting a strenuous exercise program. It may be helpful and encouraging to consult with a personal exercise trainer to get started. Choose forms of exercise that are enjoyable and that match one's abilities. For those individuals who live in climates with multiple seasons, it might be a good idea to develop ways to get exercise in each season: swimming in summer, skiing in winter, hiking in fall, and biking in spring. Vigorous exercise stimulates the release of endorphins, the body's natural opiates. This is a healthy "high," unless exercise addiction has been a problem.

Spiritual health and development will also need attention for a balanced perspective on life. Embracing one's spirituality can be a very rewarding experience.

 Question

What is spiritual direction?
Spiritual direction is the practice of helping another on his spiritual journey. A legitimate spiritual director will have training on guidance and ethics. Spiritual directors can be from any faith background. They do not provide counseling, therapy, or give advice.

Spiritual growth and development is often encouraged in some form in twelve-step groups. Many recovering addicts have found this to be an invaluable source of encouragement and inspiration. There are many avenues to spiritual growth. Reading holy writings, praying, meditating, listening to inspirational messages, and reading inspirational books are all ways that many have found helpful.

 Fact

Good self-care requires a plan for dealing with cravings should they occur. Cravings are strong mental and physical urges to engage in one's addiction. Although they lessen with time and abstinence, cravings can be reignited with a slip or relapse. Even memories of using days can trigger cravings. Cravings are one of the greatest obstacles to recovery.

Personal Growth

Personal growth is exploring the unknown in one's life as well as further refining and developing existing skills and interests. Don't let this be frightening. Yes, personal growth does require taking some risks. However, nothing compares to the risk of being involved in addictions. As always, strive to maintain a balanced approach to personal growth. This may mean trying something new physically, mentally, and spiritually. Learn a new sport, take a course studying a new subject, try a new approach to spiritual growth. Personal growth can be a great adventure, something to look forward to with anticipation and delight. Again, take it slowly, especially at first. Enjoy the process as well as the result. Try one new thing at a time, savor it fully before moving on to the next thing. Consider this: to avoid personal growth is to leave a vacuum that may make old addictive behaviors attractive again. Boredom is a dangerous enemy when it comes to recovery.

Meaningful Work and Passionate Play

When in the midst of addictive behaviors, it may have been difficult or impossible to hold down a satisfactory job. Coworkers may have been co-participants in addictive behaviors. Recovery provides an excellent reason to re-evaluate one's job satisfaction. How can a recovering addict determine if a new job would be a smart move?

- Does your current job provide a recovery-friendly environment?
- Are there triggers associated with your current job, coworkers, and so forth that might jeopardize recovery?
- Does your current job have adequate benefits for treatment and recovery needs?
- Can you be honest about addictions and recovery at your current job without fear of being fired, denied promotions, or denied opportunities?
- Is job satisfaction present with your current employment?
- Are there opportunities for personal and career growth?
- Will your current job fit in with your vision of a recovering future?

If the answer to many of these questions is no, then it's time to move forward in a different career direction. One of the secrets to successful recovery is finding satisfaction in something other than addictions. Having a career that is challenging and rewarding and that provides opportunities to give back to society in a meaningful way is an excellent way to displace a life of addictions. If a career change seems in order, see a career counselor, attend a vocational rehabilitation program, or check in with a college guidance counselor to help get ideas and direction.

Essential

In considering a career change, keep in mind that goals need to be realistic in light of one's talents, skills, training, and opportunities. Unrealistic expectations for one's career can lead to frustration, can generate negative emotions, and ultimately, can jeopardize one's recovery. Research the situation so that, with hard work, goals are reachable.

Having fun without having to worry about the consequences may have been missing from your life for a long time while addictions were in control. In recovery, it's time to play and play with passion! There will be no hangovers, no blackouts, and no fears of arrest to darken one's fun. For some recovering addicts, there may be feelings of confusion and a sense of being lost related to play. Healthy playtime may never have been a part of the picture. Don't be afraid of learning how to play. Don't allow age, career, negative emotions, shame over the past, or any other obstacle to negate one's need and right to play. Learn new games, try out fun new activities, take lessons if need be, but engage wholeheartedly in play. Again, play is about replacing addictions with a more meaningful and satisfying activity. Not only is it fun to play, but it's a protection against slips and relapses. The only thing to keep in mind is balance. Satisfying work and passionate play are to balance one another. Recovering addicts must always be watchful that life doesn't become lopsided in any one direction, even if that direction is a good one.

Making Room for Therapy

Psychotherapy may be necessary for some time to come. It can take months to years before recovery becomes one's new lifestyle, the default position. Depending on the severity of the addictions, damage to one's emotional and psychological health and damage to one's relationships may need considerable time to repair. The further along one goes into recovery, the more difficult it might be to continue the work on old issues. One would rather forget and avoid the painful past. Excuses may easily arise to justify dropping out of therapy. It's too expensive, it takes too much time from work and family, the medications are enough, and/or it's too hard. Resist these urges.

 Alert

It may be a temptation to stop psychotherapy when one begins to experience the relief and joy of recovery. This doesn't mean that the work of therapy is over. There may still be underlying or past issues that contributed to one's addiction that are not completely resolved. To terminate therapy prematurely may put one's recovery at risk.

Thoroughly examining and resolving the problems that may have contributed to one's addictions will be well worth the effort in the end. Particularly if there are co-occurring mental health problems, continuing in therapy is essential for recovery. Consult with one's therapist about the issues that would be helpful to address, effective interventions, and the signs of progress. Ideally, termination of therapy should occur with the mutual agreement of both the recovering addict and the therapist.

Developing Satisfying Relationships

A recovering addict may deeply desire satisfying relationships but be completely at a loss in knowing how to develop them. The recovering addict has a long history of using manipulation, lies, deception, and avoidance in managing relationships. Relationships built on those qualities are far from satisfying.

 Question

Is it healthy for two people in recovery to become romantically involved?
There are advantages and disadvantages to a relationship involving two recovering addicts. While there will be a unique understanding about the other's background, if one slips or relapses, the other might be at greater risk to do the same. If both are involved in good, healthy, solid recovery, it could be a very satisfying union. Proceed with caution.

What should a recovering addict who has never experienced a healthy relationship look for? Here are some guidelines.

- Each person has a realistic perception of the other.
- Each person takes responsibility for his or her own growth and recovery.
- Each person can communicate in an assertive, adult manner.
- Each person is willing to engage in constructive problem-solving when needed.
- Each person has a fulfilling life in his or her own right.
- Each person is capable of good self-care as well as good other-care.
- Each person can be comfortable either alone or with others.
- Each person is willing to accept and honor differences in the other.

Sounds wonderful, doesn't it? It is. However, most healthy relationships are works in progress. The point is, healthy and satisfying relationships aspire to these guidelines and are well on the way to reaching them. Healthy relationships can see differences as assets, providing variety and flavor rather than engendering conflict and criticism. A healthy friend is supportive, encouraging, and kind, but also honest. He will not shy away from the truth, even if the other doesn't want to hear it. The other's welfare is more important than being right or keeping interactions going smoothly. This type of relationship is a tremendous blessing for the recovering addict.

Leave the Past Behind and Look to the Future

It's time for the recovering addict and his family to turn the corner for good. Although it may seem impossible to leave the past behind, it's necessary for recovery.

Leaving the past behind is not about forgetting. Forgetting what one has experienced negates and disrespects what one learned from the experience. Memories also serve to reinforce the need to move into a future of recovery. Memories of the past pain, difficult consequences, lost relationships, and poor health can motivate one to avoid repetition. Leaving the past behind implies that it has lost its power to influence the future in a negative way. Past mistakes are no longer the model or pattern for future behavior. The recovering addict's perception of herself is no longer dependent on past problems and mistakes. She is free to grow and mature into the person she desires to become.

Forgiveness provides the freedom to move into the future. For the recovering addict, forgiveness must be both requested and received. The recovering addict must ask for forgiveness from those he's damaged through his addictions. He must also ask for forgiveness from himself. Asking for forgiveness is not enough—it's only half of the equation. Receiving forgiveness from others and oneself may be the most difficult part of this interaction. The recovering addict may feel unworthy, undeserving, and ashamed. Hanging onto these negative feelings will keep him trapped between the past and the future.

 Fact

> Recovery from addictions is possible! The recovering addict must resist all input that says otherwise. Hope and a future are based on the belief that recovery can be achieved with hard work and perseverance. Recovery will change the addict's life in ways she never thought possible. Invite recovery and welcome it wholeheartedly when it arrives!

Acceptance of forgiveness is necessary to prepare the recovering addict for future growth. To be forgiven is a gift to be gratefully welcomed. To look forward to the future is to envision possibilities and to work at making those possibilities reality. No one knows what challenges the future may present. However, the recovering addict has gained knowledge, skills, and maturity through her recovery efforts. Those assets will provide her with the confidence and ability to handle future challenges. It is very important that the recovering addict give herself permission to enjoy the future, to look forward to it, and to share it willingly with others. Recovery is a blessed event and achievement that deserves celebration!

Resources

Websites

Addiction Recovery Basics
www.addictionrecoverybasics.com

Addiction Recovery Skills and Coping Strategies
www.addictionsandrecovery.org/recovery-skills.htm

Gamblers Anonymous
www.gamblersanonymous.org

Food Pyramid
www.mypyramid.gov

Home Box Office project focusing on addictions
www.hbo.com/addiction

Internet Addiction
www.virtual-addiction.com

Join Together (a project of the Boston University School of Public Health)
www.jointogether.org

Love Addicts Anonymous
www.loveaddicts.org

Mothers Against Drunk Driving (MADD)
www.madd.org

Online Gambling Myths & Facts
www.onlinegamblingmythsandfacts.com

National Association for Children of Alcoholics (NACoA)
www.nacoa.net

National Eating Disorders
www.nationaleatingdisorders.org

National Council on Problem Gambling
www.ncpgambling.org

National Institute on Alcohol Abuse and Alcoholism (NIAAA)
www.niaaa.nih.gov

National Council on Alcoholism and Drug Dependence (NCADD)
www.ncadd.org

National Institute on Drug Abuse (NIDA)
www.nida.nih.gov

Office of National Drug Control Policy (ONDCP)
www.whitehousedrugpolicy.gov

Online Gamers Anonymous
www.olganon.org

Partnership for a Drug-Free America
www.drugfree.org

Relationship Addiction
www.relationshipaddict.com

Safe Families—Keeping Children Safe Online
www.safefamilies.org

Sexual Recovery Institute
www.sexualrecovery.com

The Addiction Recovery Guide
www.addictionrecoveryguide.org

Workaholics Anonymous
www.workaholics-anonymous.org

Books

Beck, Aaron T., Wright, Fred D., Newman, Cory F., & Liese, Bruce S. *Cognitive Therapy of Substance Abuse* (New York, London: The Guilford Press, 1993).

Carnes, Patrick, Delmonico, David L., Griffin, Elizabeth, & Moriarity, Joseph M. *In the Shadows of the Net: Breaking Free of Compulsive Online Sexual Behavior* (Center City, MN: Hazelden, 2001).

Colvin, Rod. *Prescription Drug Addiction: The Hidden Epidemic* (Omaha, NE: Addicus Books, 2002).

Coombs, Robert Holman & Howatt, William A. *The Addiction Counselor's Desk Reference* (Hoboken, NJ: John Wiley & Sons, 2005).

Daley, Dennis C. *Addiction and Mood Disorders* (New York: Oxford University Press, 2006).

DiClemente, Carlo C. *Addiction and Change: How Addictions Develop and Addicted People Recover* (New York, London: The Guildford Press, 2003).

Gwinnell, Esther & Adamec, Christine. *The Encyclopedia of Addictions and Addictive Behaviors* (New York: Facts on File, 2006).

Halpern, Howard M. *How to Break Your Addiction to a Person* (New York: Bantam Books, 2004).

Howard, Pierce J. *The Owner's Manual for the Brain: Everyday Applications from Mind-Brain Research, 3d ed.* (Austin, TX: Bard Press, 2006).

Katherine, Anne. *Anatomy of a Food Addiction* (New York: Simon and Schuster, 1991).

Krestan, Jo-Ann (ed.). *Bridges to Recovery: Addiction, Family Therapy, and Multicultural Treatment* (New York: The Free Press, 2000).

L., Elisabeth. *Twelve Steps for Overeaters* (San Francisco: Harper & Row, 1988).

Lee, Steven J. *Overcoming Crystal Meth Addiction: An Essential Guide to Getting Clean* (New York: Marlowe & Company, 2006).

Marohn, Stephanie. *The Natural Medicine Guide to Addiction* (Charlottesville, VA: Hampton Roads Publishing Company, 2004).

Mellody, Pia. *Facing Love Addiction* (San Francisco: HarperSanFrancisco, 1992).

Mooney, Al J., Eisenberg, Arlene, & Eisenberg, Howard. *The Recovery Book* (New York: Workman Publishing, 1992).

Nakken, Craig. *Reclaim Your Family from Addiction: How Couples and Families Recover Love and Meaning* (Center City, MN: Hazelden, 2000).

Nakken, Craig. *The Addictive Personality: Understanding the Addictive Process and Compulsive Behavior* (Center City, MN: Hazelden, 1996).

Paul, Pamela. *Pornified: How Pornography Is Damaging Our Lives, Our Relationships, and Our Families* (New York: Henry Holt and Company, 2005).

Prentiss, Chris. *The Alcoholism and Addiction Cure: A Holistic Approach to Total Recovery* (Los Angeles: Power Press, 2006).

Skinner, Kevin B. *Treating Pornography Addiction: The Essential Tools for Recovery* (Provo, UT: GrowthClimate, Inc., 2005).

Solomon, Melanie. *AA Not the Only Way: Your One Stop Resource Guide to 12-Step Alternatives* (Anchorage, AK: Capalo Press, 2005).

Waite, Terry R. *Plugged In: A Clinician's and Families' Guide to Online Video Game Addiction* (Baltimore, MD: PublishAmerica, 2007).

Organizations/Support Groups

Al-Anon Family Group Headquarters
(888) 425-2666

www.al-anon.alateen.org

Alcoholics Anonymous (A.A.) World Services
(212) 870-3400

www.aa.org

The Department of Health and Human Sevices Substance Abuse and Mental Health Sevices Administration's (SAMHSA's) Center for Substance Abuse Prevention (CSAP)
(800)729-6686

http://prevention.samhsa.gov

Codependents of Sex Addicts (COSA)
National Service Organization

P.O. Box 14537

Minneapolis, MN 55414

www.cosa-recovery.org

Dual Diagnosis Recovery Network (DRN)
(877) 345-3357

http://dualdiagnosis.org/resource/ddrn

Families Anonymous, Inc. (FA)
P.O. Box 3475

Culver City, CA 90231-3475

(800) 736-9805

www.familiesanonymous.org

Nar-Anon Family Group
P.O. Box 2562

Palos Verdes Peninsula, CA 90274

(310) 547-5800

http://nar-anon.org

National Alliance for the Mentally Ill (NAMI)
Colonial Place Three
2107 Wilson Blvd., Suite 300
Arlington, VA 22201-3042
(800) 950-NAMI
www.nami.org

National Clearinghouse for Alcohol and Drug Information (NCADI)
11426-28 Rockville Pike, Suite 200
Rockville, MD 20847-2345
(800) 729-6686
www.ncadi.samhsa.gov

National Council on Problem Gambling
(800) 522-4700
www.ncpgambling.org

National Eating Disorders Association
(800) 931-2237
www.nationaleatingdisorders.org

Substance Abuse and Mental Health Services Administration (SAMHSA)
U.S. Department of Health and Human Services (DHHS)
5600 Fishers Lane
Parklawn Building, Suite 13C-05
Rockville, MD 20857
www.samhsa.gov

Substance Abuse Treatment Facility Locator
(800) 662-4357
www.findtreatment.samhsa.gov

Street Names and Slang Associated with Substance Addiction

Abandominiums abandoned row houses where drugs are used

Abe $5 worth of drugs

A-bomb marijuana cigarette with heroin or opium

AC/DC codeine cough syrup

Acapulco gold marijuana from S. W. Mexico

Acid LSD

Adam MDMA, Ecstasy

AIP heroin from Afghanistan, Iran, Pakistan

Air blast inhalant

All lit up under the influence of drugs

Amp amphetamine

Angel dust PCP

Antifreeze heroin

Apache fentanyl

Apple jacks crack cocaine

Arnolds steroids

Artillery equipment for injecting drugs

Aunt Hazel heroin

Aunt Mary marijuana

Aunt Nora cocaine

Author doctor who writes illegal prescriptions

Baby habit occasional use of drugs

Babysit guide someone through his first drug experience

Backjack inject opium, to inject a drug

Bad seed marijuana combined with peyote, heroin

Bag man person who transports money or drugs

Bagging using inhalants

---

*This is a sampling of 2,300 street terms related to drugs or drug activity. The Office of National Drug Control Policy collected this information from law enforcement personnel, health care professionals, and others. The full list was published in May 2006 and may be found on the web at *www.whitehousedrugpolicy.gov*.

Banana split combination of 2C-B (Nexus) with other illicit substances such as LSD

Bank bandit pills depressants

Barbies depressants

Bart Simpson heroin

Baseball crack cocaine

Bathtub crank poor quality methamphetamine

Batted out apprehended by the law

Bazooka cocaine; combination of crack and marijuana; coca paste and marijuana

Beam me up Scottie cocaine combined with PCP

Beannies methamphetamines

Beat artist person selling bogus drugs

Beavis & Butthead LSD

Bed bugs fellow addicts

Belushi combination of cocaine and heroin

Bender drug party

Bikers coffee methamphetamine and coffee

Biscuit 50 rocks of crack

Bite one's lips smoke marijuana

Black eagle heroin

Black gold high-potency marijuana

Black hole the depressant high associated with ketamine

Blow cocaine

Blue devils depressants

Blue kisses MDMA

Blue mollies amphetamine

Blue vials LSD

Brain ticklers amphetamine

Buddha potent marijuana spiked with opium

Buttons mescaline

Cactus mescaline

Cadillac cocaine, PCP

Cafeteria-style use using a combination of different club drugs

Candy sticks marijuana cigarettes laced with powdered cocaine

Candyman drug supplier

Cartwheels amphetamine

Casper the ghost crack cocaine

Catnip marijuana cigarette

Caviar combination of cocaine and marijuana

Champagne combination of cocaine and marijuana

Channel vein into which a drug is injected

Chasing the tiger smoking heroin

Cheese mix of ground-up cold medicine and a small amount of heroin

China town fentanyl

Cloud nine crack cocaine or MDMA

Cocoa puff to smoke cocaine and marijuana

Coffee LSD

Come home end a "trip" from LSD

Comic book LSD

Cookies crack cocaine

Cotton OxyContin

Courage pills heroin, depressants

Cracker jack crack smoker

Crap low quality heroin

Crystal glass crystal shards of methamphetamine

Cubes marijuana tablets, crack cocaine

Dance fever fentanyl

Dead president heroin

Detroit pink PCP

Devil's dust PCP

Dew marijuana

Dice crack cocaine

Dinosaurs populations of heroin users in their forties and fifties

Disco pellet stimulant

Do a line to inhale cocaine

Dog food heroin

Domino amphetamine

Double cross amphetamine

Dr. Feelgood heroin

Dragon rock mixture of heroin and crack

Dream stick opium

Dummy dust PCP

Easy lay GHB

E-bombs MDMA

Eightball crack mixed with heroin

Electric Kool Aid LSD

Embalming fluid PCP

Explorers club group of LSD users

Eye opener crack; amphetamine

Factory place where drugs are packaged, diluted, or manufactured

Fall arrested

Fantasia dimethyltryptamine

Fast white lady powder cocaine

Felix the Cat LSD

Finger marijuana cigarette

Fire crack and methamphetamine

Fish scales crack cocaine

Fizzies methadone

Flakes PCP

Flea powder low purity heroin

Fleece counterfeit crack cocaine

Flower marijuana

Footballs amphetamine

Forget me drug Rohypnol

Four leaf clover MDMA

Freebase to smoke cocaine

French fries crack cocaine

Frisco special cocaine, heroin, and LSD

Galloping horse heroin

Gangster person who uses or manufactures methamphetamine

Garbage inferior quality marijuana; low quality heroin

Geek crack mixed with marijuana

Geezer to inject a drug

Georgia home boy (GHB) gamma hydroxybutyric acid, a synthetic depressant

Get a gift obtain drugs

Getting roached using Rohypnol

Ghost LSD

Giggle weed marijuana

Girlfriend cocaine

Glass heroin; amphetamine; hypodermic needle; methamphetamine

Go on a sleigh ride to inhale cocaine

Goat heroin

Golden dragon LSD

Golf balls depressants

Good horse heroin

Gorilla pills depressants

Graduate completely stop using drugs; or progress to stronger drugs

Grasshopper marijuana

Green tea PCP

Groceries crack cocaine

Gum opium

Gym candy steroids

Haircut marijuana

Hamburger helper crack cocaine

Happy dust cocaine

Hard candy heroin

Hawaiian very high potency marijuana

Hawkers individuals who walk through nightclubs announcing the availability of drugs

Heaven & Hell PCP

Henpecking searching on hands and knees for crack

Henry VIII cocaine

Hero of the underworld heroin

Hillbilly heroin OxyContin

Hitch up the reindeers to inhale cocaine

Hog PCP

Honey currency

Horse heroin

Hotcakes crack cocaine

Hustle attempt to obtain drug customers

Ice cocaine; crack cocaine; smokable methamphetamine; PCP

Ice cream habit occasional use of drugs

Idiot pills depressants

Jack steal someone else's drugs

Jane marijuana

Jellies combination of depressants and MDMA

Jelly bean amphetamine; depressants

Jet fuel PCP; methamphetamine

Jim Jones marijuana laced with cocaine and PCP

Joy juice depressants

Juggler teen-aged street dealer

Ju-ju marijuana cigarette

Junkie addict

Kangaroo crack

Karo codeine cough syrup

K-hole periods of ketamine-induced confusion; the depressant high of ketamine

Kicker OxyContin

Kiddie dope prescription drugs

King Kong pills depressants

Kissing the exchange of plastic wrapped rocks (crack) by kissing or mouth to mouth transfer

Klingons crack addicts

Lace cocaine and marijuana

Laughing grass marijuana

Leapers amphetamine

Lemonade heroin; poor quality drugs

Lid poppers amphetamine

Lightning amphetamine

Lipton tea poor quality drugs

Locker room inhalants

Loony Toons LSD

Love flipping use of mescaline and MDMA

Love pill MDMA

Loveboat combination of PCP and marijuana

Lunch money drug Rohypnol

Macaroni marijuana

Magic dust PCP

Magic mushroom psilocybin

Mainline to inject a drug

Marathon amphetamine

Marching powder cocaine

Matchbox ¼ ounce of marijuana or 6 marijuana cigarettes

Maxibolin oral steroids

Mean green PCP

Mellow yellow LSD

Mercedes MDMA

Meth monster one who has a violent reaction to methamphetamine

Mexican valium Rohypnol

Mighty Joe Young depressants

Mind detergent LSD

Miss Emma morphine

Monkey cigarette made from cocaine paste and tobacco

Moon mescaline

Moon gas inhalant

Morning wake-up first blast of crack from the pipe

Mother marijuana

Mother's little helper depressants

Nail marijuana cigarette

New Jack Swing heroin and morphine

Noise heroin

Northern lights marijuana from Canada

Nose drops liquefied heroin

Nose powder cocaine

Nuggets crack cocaine

Octane PCP laced with gasoline

On a trip under the influence of drugs

On ice in jail

Onion one ounce of crack cocaine

Optical illusions LSD

Orange bandits MDMA

Orange wedges LSD

Outerlimits crack and LSD

Oxycotton OxyContin

Oyster stew cocaine

Pack of rocks marijuana cigarette

Pancakes and syrup combination of glutethimide and codeine cough syrup

Pane LSD

Paper a dosage unit of heroin; one-tenth of a gram or less of the drug ice or methamphetamine

Paper bag container for drugs

Parachute crack and PCP smoked; heroin; smokable crack and heroin mixture

Parachute down use of MDMA after heroin

Parsley marijuana combined with PCP

Paste crack cocaine

Peace pill PCP

Peaches amphetamines

Peanut butter methamphetamine; PCP mixed with peanut butter

Pearly gates LSD

Peeper(s) MDMA user(s)

Pep pill amphetamine

Pepsi habit occasional use of drugs

Perp fake crack made of candle wax and baking soda

Piggybacking simultaneous injection of two drugs

Pink elephant methamphetamine

Pink panther MDMA

Pony crack cocaine

Poor man's heroin Talwin and Ritalin combination is injected and produces an effect similar to the effect of heroin mixed with cocaine

Potato chips crack cut with benzocaine

Puff the dragon smoking marijuana

Pumpers steroids

Purple rain PCP

Quarter bag $25 worth of drugs

Quartz smokable methamphetamine

Queen Ann's lace marijuana

Quicksilver isobutyl nitrite; inhalants

Racehorse Charlie cocaine; heroin

Rainbows depressants

Raspberry female who trades sex for crack or money to buy crack

Rave all-night dance parties frequently designed to enhance a hallucinogenic experience through music and lights

Raw hide heroin

Razed under the influence of drugs

Red devil MDMA

Red eagle heroin

Reefer marijuana

Reindeer dust heroin

Rest in peace crack cocaine

Rib Rohypnol; MDMA

Riding the wave under the influence of drugs

Ringer good hit of crack

Roach butt of marijuana cigarette

Road dope amphetamine

Robin's egg stimulant

Rock methamphetamine

Rocket fuel PCP

Rollers police

Rolls Royce MDMA

Roofies Rohypnol

Roses amphetamine

Ruffles Rohypnol

Runners people who sell drugs for others or who act as liaisons between sellers and buyers

Rush cocaine; isobutyl nitrite; inhalants

Salt heroin

Sam federal narcotics agent

Sandwich two layers of cocaine with a layer of heroin in the middle

Satan's secret inhalants

Schoolboy cocaine; codeine

Scissors marijuana

Scooby snacks MDMA

Score purchase drugs

Scrabble crack cocaine

Scratch money

Seeds marijuana

Serial speedballing sequencing cocaine, cough syrup, and heroin over a one- to two-day period

Server crack dealer

Seven-up crack cocaine

Sharps hypodermic needles

Sheet rocking crack and LSD

Shoot the breeze Inhale nitrous oxide

Shooting gallery place where drugs are used

Shot to the curb lost everything to crack

Shrooms psilocybin/psilocin

Silk heroin

Skag heroin

Skeegers crack-smoking prostitutes

Sketching coming down from a speed-induced high

Skunk marijuana; heroin

Slanging selling drugs

Sleigh ride cocaine

Smack heroin

Smoke houses crack houses

Smurf cigar dipped in embalming fluid

Snackies MDMA mixed with mescaline

Sniffer bag $5 bag of heroin intended for inhalation

Snotballs rubber cement rolled into balls, burned and the fumes are inhaled

Snowcone cocaine

Soda injectable cocaine

Soup crack cocaine

Space cadet crack dipped in PCP

Sparklers amphetamine

Speed crack cocaine; amphetamine; methamphetamine

Spider heroin

Splitting rolling marijuana and cocaine into a single joint

Spray inhalant

Stackers steroids

Star dust PCP

Stash place to hide drugs

Stink weed marijuana

Stove top crystal methamphetamine; methamphetamine

Strawberries depressants

Sugar cubes LSD

Swallower person used as a drug courier

Swishers cigars in which tobacco is replaced with marijuana

T.N.T. heroin; fentanyl

Tail lights LSD

Taking a cruise PCP

Tango & Cash fentanyl

Tar crack and heroin smoked together

Taxing price paid to enter a crackhouse; charging more per vial depending on race of customer; charging if not a regular customer

Tea party to smoke marijuana

Teeth cocaine; crack cocaine

Tester individual who is given a drug early in the day by a dealer and then spreads the word about the drug

Thai sticks bundles of marijuana soaked in hashish oil; marijuana buds bound on short sections of bamboo

Thirst monster crack smoker

Thoroughbred drug dealer who sells pure narcotics

Tina methamphetamine; crystal methamphetamine

Tissue crack cocaine

Toilet water inhalants

Tooties depressants

Tootsie roll heroin

Torch cooking smoking cocaine base by using a propane or butane torch as a source of flame

Tornado crack cocaine

Torpedo marijuana and crack

Touter person who stands on the street and advertises a drug

Toys opium

Tracks row of needle marks on a person

Train heroin

Travel agent LSD supplier

Triple crowns MDMA

Trippin' high on drugs

Truck drivers amphetamine

Turf place where drugs are sold

Turkey cocaine; amphetamine

Turned on introduced to drugs; under the influence

Tweaker crack user looking for drugs on the floor after a police raid

Twinkie crack cocaine

Twist marijuana cigarette

Ultimate crack cocaine

Uncle Milty depressants

Uppers amphetamine

Uptown powder cocaine

Viper marijuana smoker

Vitamin K ketamine

Vitamin R Ritalin

Vodka acid LSD

Wafers MDMA

Waffle dust combination of MDMA and amphetamine

Wasted under the influence of drugs; murdered

Watercolors LSD

Wedding bells LSD

Weight trainers steroids

Weightless high on crack

Wet sticks marijuana combined with PCP and formaldehyde

Wheat marijuana

Whiffledust amphetamine; MDMA

White cloud smoke that collects in bottom of crack pipe; crack smoke

White dove MDMA

White ghost crack cocaine

White lightening LSD

Wicked a potent brand of heroin

Wicky stick PCP, marijuana, and crack

Window glass LSD

Witch cocaine; heroin

Wolfies Rohypnol

Woolas cigarettes laced with cocaine; crack sprinkled on marijuana cigarette

Working selling crack

Working man's cocaine methamphetamine

Wrecking crew crack cocaine

Yahoo crack cocaine

Yellow LSD; depressants

Yellow fever PCP

Yellow jackets depressants; methamphetamine

Ying Yang LSD

Zen LSD

Zip cocaine

Zombie PCP; heavy user of drugs

Zulu bogus crack

INDEX

Acamprosate (Campral), 203–4
Acupuncture, 210
Addictionologist, 22–23, 198
Addiction(s). *See also specific types*
  affect of, on family members,
    133–34, 259–73
  biological effects of, 6–8
  brain chemistry and, 6–7,
    13–14, 30–31
  causes of, 27–38
  costs of, 191–92, 199
  disease model of, 20–21, 27–28, 46
  emotional effects of, 8–10
  vs. impulsive behavior, 121–23
  multiple, 8, 91, 138
  nature of, 1–14
  psychological effects of, 10–14
  risk factors for, 15–19
  seeking help for, 48
  symptoms of, 19–21
Addiction vaccines, 93, 205
Addictive behaviors, recognizing, 23–25
Addictive personality, 37–38
Addictive substances. *See* Drugs
Addicts
  approaching, about addiction,
    23–25, 60–61, 76–78, 90–91, 105–6,
    134, 145–46, 185–86, 199–200
  denial by, 25–26, 77, 188–91
Adolescents. *See also* Youth
  development of addictions in, x, 31
  gambling addiction and, 137
  influences on, 16–18
  relapse in, 234
  smoking by, 82, 83, 85
Advertising, 39–41
Alcohol
  affect on women vs. men, 57–59
  mental health problems and, 53
  mixing with medications, 102
  mood effects of, 56–57
  physiological effects of, 51–52
  social drinking of, 54–56
Alcohol advertising, 40
Alcoholics Anonymous (A.A.),
  28, 62–63, 216, 227
Alcoholism

brain and, 49–51
as co-addiction, 138
defined, 49–54
development of, 4
as disease, 27–28
dry drunks and, 63–64
genetic factors in, 28–29, 53–54
medications for treating, 203–5
negative effects of, 2
recovery from, 61–62
signs and symptoms of, 59–60
talking to loved one about, 60–61
twelve-step programs for, 62–63
Alcohol poisoning, 52
Alcopop, 44
Alternative treatment options,
  92, 209–16
Amotivational syndrome, 67
Amphetamines, 73
Amygdala, 6, 13, 43, 163–64, 165
Androgens, 172
Anger, 9
Anhedonia, 9
Animal therapy, 216
Anonymity, 184–85
Antabuse (disulfiram), 62, 204
Antiandrogens, 172
Anxiety, 23, 50, 53, 56, 110, 153
Aromatherapy, 211–12
Attention Deficit Hyperactivity
  Disorder (ADHD), 103, 178
Availability, of substances, 31–32
Ayurveda, 215

Baclofen, 208
Bad habits, 15–16
Beecher, Lyman, 28
Beer, 4
Behavioral addictions
  effect of, on family members, 133–34
  exercise, 126–29
  impulsive behavior vs.
    addiction, 121–23
  seeking help for, 134–35
  shoplifting, 131–33
  shopping/spending, 123–26
  signs of, 120–21

talking to loved one about, 134
work, 129–31
Behavioral therapy, for nicotine
addiction, 91–92
Beta-endorphins, 85
Binge-eating disorder, 109, 118
Biofeedback, 209–10
Biological effects, 6–8
Biological factors
in addiction, 30–31
in gambling addiction, 137–38
in love addiction, 151–52
in sex addiction, 156–57
Bipolar disorder, 56–57
Blood alcohol concentration (BAC), 55
Body language, 264
Boredom, 227
Brain
affect of childhood trauma on, 33
affect of drugs on, 72–74
alcohol and the, 49–51, 56
gambling addiction and the, 137–38
love addiction and, 151
nicotine and the, 84–86
pornography addiction and, 163–65
video games and the, 178–79
Brain chemistry, 6–7, 13–14, 30–31.
See also Neurotransmitters
Brain structures, 12, 13, 43
Brain waves, 179, 210
Buprenorphine, 107, 206–7
Buproprion (Zyban or Wellbutrin), 205–6
Buspirone (Buspar), 206

Caffeine, 69
Calcium, 277
Campral (acamprosate), 203–4
Cancer, 52, 58, 86
Cannabinoids, 67, 73
Casinos, 40–41, 136, 141–42
Causes, 27–38
Celebrity influences, 44–46
Cell phone addiction, 180–82
Central nervous system (CNS)
depressants, 66–67, 74,
78–79, 96, 102–3
Cerebral cortex, 12, 13
Chantix (varenicline), 206
Chat room addiction, 159–60
Child pornography, 170–71

Children. See also Youth
born to nicotine-addicted mothers, 88
of gambling addicts, 145
learned behavior in, 33–35
parenting issues and, 256–57
pornography and, 167–68
risk factors for, 19
Chocolate, 114
Cigarette smoking. See
Nicotine addiction
Club drugs, 70
Cocaine, 73, 207–8
Cognitive-behavioral therapy
(CBT), 219–22
Cognitive functioning, 13–14
Communication, 263–65
Community, restoring
credibility in, 257–58
Community involvement, 32–33
Community resources, 228–29
Compulsive behaviors, x, 5
Compulsive buying, 123–26
Conflicts, 265–67
Confrontations, 77
Constructive fighting, 265–67
Cortisol, 85
CRAFT (Community Reinforcement
and Family Training), 199–200
Cravings, 6, 113
Creative arts therapies, 215
CREB (cyclic AMP response
element-binding protein), 50
Credibility, 257–58
Criminal activities, 8, 16, 32–33, 75–76
Cultural differences, 46–47
Curiosity, 41–43
Cybersex, 157–59

Daily thought records (DTRs), 222
D.A.R.E. (Drug Abuse Resistance
Education), 18
Date-rape drugs, 70, 72
Debt, 244–46
Defense mechanisms, 188–91
Denial, 10–11, 25–26, 77, 188–91
Dependence. See Substance dependence
Depressants, 66–67, 74, 78–79, 96, 102–3
Depression, 23, 50, 53, 56–57, 84, 153
Designer drugs, x, 66, 74–75
Desipramine (Norpramin), 207

Detoxification, 201–02
Digestive system, 51–52
Disappointment, 9
Disease model, 20–21, 27–28, 46
Distorted thinking, 23, 36–37, 219–20
Disulfiram (Antabuse), 62, 204
Dopamine
    addiction and, 6–7, 18, 30–31, 43
    affect of drugs on, 70–73, 84–86, 103
    love addiction and, 151
    pleasure pathway, 30–31, 72–73
Drink serving size, 55
Drug-related crimes, 75–76
Drugs. See also Medications;
    specific drugs
    body's reaction to, 72–74
    categories of, 65–69
    common, for abuse, 70–72
    designer, x, 66, 74–75
    prescription, 95–107
Drug-test kits, 23
Dry drunks, 63–64
Dual diagnosis, xi, 56

Eating disorders, 109, 117, 127.
    See also Food addiction
e-cards, 223
Ecstasy (MDMA), 70–72, 74–75
Elderly, 97–98
Emotional boundaries, 263
Emotions
    addiction and, 8–10, 18–19, 109–10
    dealing with difficult, 261–63
Employers/employment issues,
    198–99, 246–49, 279–80
Enabling, 259–60
Endorphins, 114, 127
Entertainment, addiction and, 25,
    40, 42, 45, 136–37, 165–68
Environmental factors, 17–18, 31–33, 139
e-pharmacies, 99
Ethnic differences, 46–47
Exercise addiction, 126–29
External pressures, 47–48

Faith-based treatment programs, 216–17
Family history, 15
Family members/relationships
    affect of addiction on, 133–34, 259–73
    communication among, 263–65

constructive fighting and, 265–67
difficult emotions in, 261–63
enabling by, 259–60
establishing new and healthy, 272–73
financial hardships and, 270–71
learned behavior and, 33–35
recovery and, 249–51
role reversals in, 267–70
trust building in, 271–72
Fast food, 115–16
Fear, 9
Fetal alcohol syndrome (FAS), 58
Financial problems, 243–46, 270–71
Flashbacks, 75
Fluoxetine (Prozac), 206
Food addiction
    behavioral contributions to, 109–11
    fast food and, 115–16
    overview of, 108–09
    signs of, 109
    societal pressures and, 111–12
    talking to loved one about, 116–18
    treatment options for, 118–19
    types of food for, 112–14
Forgiveness, 283–84
Friendships, 239–40, 251–52
Funitrazepam (Rohypnol), 72

GABA (gamma-aminobutyric
    acid), 49–50, 74, 102
Gabapentin (Gabitrol), 208
Gambling
    Internet, 144
    legalized, 141–44
    social costs of, 142–43
Gambling addiction
    biology of, 137–38
    effects of, on family members, 144–45
    phases of, 138–39
    signs of, 140–41
    talking to loved one about, 145–46
    treatment options for, 146–47
Gamma hydroxybutyrate (GHB), 72
Gamma-vinyl-GABA (GVG), 208
Gastritis, 51–52
Genetic factors, 15, 20, 28–30, 53–54, 137
Glutamate, 13–14, 49–50, 73–74
Grandiose thinking, 11–12
Gray market, 141
Guided imagery, 214, 221

Hallucinogens, 67–68, 73–74
Harrison Anti-Narcotic Act, 28–29
Hashish, 67, 74
Health consequences
    of addictions, 7–8, 51–52
    of nicotine, 86–87
    of secondhand smoke, 88–89
Heart problems, 52, 86
Herbal therapy, 213
Heroin addiction, 206–8
High-risk situations, 237–39
Hippocampus, 13, 43
HIV/AIDS, 8
Homeopathy, 212
Household issues, 249–51
Hurt, 9–10
Huss, Magnus, 28
Hypertension, 52
Hypnosis, 211
Hypoglycemia, 214
Hypothalamus, 108

Immune system, 52, 86
Impulse-control disorders, 121–23, 138
Inhalants, 7, 75
Insurance coverage, for
    treatment, 192–94
Internet
    addiction to, 182–84
    chat room addiction, 159–60
    cybersex, 157–59
    radio programs, 222
    scams, 185
Internet gambling, 144

Job issues, 246–49, 279–80

Korsakoff's syndrome, 13

Learning/learned behavior, 13–14, 33–35
Levo-Alpha Acetyl Methadol
    (LAAM), 207
Life balance, 274–84
Life expectancy, 54
Lithium, 147
Love addiction, 148–53
Lying, 218, 250

Male sexuality, 163–65
MAO (monoamine oxidase), 50

Marijuana, 32, 67, 73, 74
MDMA (Ecstasy), 70, 71–72, 74–75
Medications. *See also* Prescription
    drugs; *specific types*
    mixing, 53, 56, 102, 104
    for nicotine addiction, 93–94
    over-the-counter (OTC), 96, 102, 104
    for treating addictions, xi, 61–62,
        93–94, 172–73, 203–9
Meditation, 214
Memory, 13–14
Men, affect of alcohol on, 57–59
Mental health disorders, xi,
    35–36, 38, 53, 87–88, 122
Mental health parity, 192–93
Mental health professionals, 197–98
Methadone, 107, 207
Methamphetamines, 32, 70–71
Mind-body-spirit connection, 274–75
Modafinil (Provigil), 208
Mood, alcohol's effects on, 56–57
Morphine derivatives, 68
Motivational interviewing, 77–78
Movies, 41–42
Multiple addictions, 8, 91, 138

Naltrexone, 107, 147, 204
Nefazodone (Serzone), 204
Negative self-talk, 37
Neuroadaptation, 5
Neurotransmitters. *See also*
    specific neurotransmitters
    addiction and, 6–7, 18
    affect of drugs on, 72–74,
        84–86, 103–4
    alcohol and, 49–50, 57
    gambling and, 137–38
    love addiction and, 151–52
Nicotine, 69, 73, 81, 84–87
Nicotine addiction
    difficulty of overcoming, 89–90
    medications for treating, 205–06
    overview of, 81–84
    psychological component of, 87–88
    signs and symptoms of, 81–82
    talking to loved one about, 90–91
    treatment options for, 91–94
Nicotine poisoning, 87
Nicotine replacement treatments, 93,
    205

NMDA (N-methyl-D-aspartate),
49–50, 73
Nocaine, 208
Norepineprhine, 103, 137, 151
Norpramin (desipramine), 207
Nutrition, 213–14

Obesity, 116
Obsessive thinking, 11
Online support groups, 222–23
Opiates
abuse of prescription, 100–101
addiction to, 68, 73, 74, 78, 95
treatment for addiction to, 107
Osteoporosis, 52
Outdoor therapy, 215–16
Outpatient treatment programs,
195–96
Overeaters Anonymous (OA), 119
Overeating. See Food addiction
Over-the-counter (OTC)
medications, 96, 102, 104
OxyContin, 101

Pain medications, 98, 100–101
Pancrease, 52
Paraphilias, 155–56
Parenting issues, 16, 256–57
Past, leaving behind the, 283–84
Peer pressure, x, 16–17, 43–44
Personal growth, 278–79
Pet therapy, 216
Phenylethylamine (PEA), 151
Physical health, 274–78
Physiological effects, 51–52, 84–87
Pitfalls, 254–56
Placebo effect, 212
Playtime, 280–81
Pleasure circuit, 6, 9, 13–14,
30–31, 43, 72–73
Pornography addiction
beginnings of, 42–43
effects of, on relationships, 168–70
vs. entertainment, 165–68
legal implications of, 170–71
male sexuality and, 163–65
partner support and, 173
signs of, 166–67
treatment for, 171–73
Positive reinforcement, 34–35

Positive self-talk, 234–35
Prefrontal cortex, 30
Pregnancy, 56, 58, 86, 88
Premature aging, 50, 86
Prescription drug addiction
identifying, 99–100
medications for treating, 206–7
risk for, 96–99
talking to loved one about, 105–6
treatment for, 106–7
Prescription drugs
commonly abused, 100–104
measures to obtain, 104–5
overview of, 95–96
Procrastination, 254–56
Provigil (modafinil), 208
Prozac (fluoxetine), 206
Psychiatric disorders, xi, 35–36,
38, 53, 87–88, 122
Psychological effects, of addiction, 10–14
Psychological factors, 35–37, 87–88
Psychotherapy, 281
Public health model, 32

Qi, 209

Reactive attachment disorder, 149–50
Recovery. See also Relapse prevention
accountability and, 260
challenges to, 13
changing thinking patterns for, 219–22
community resources for, 228–29
of family relationships, 259–73
life balance and, 274–84
process of, 79–80, 218–19, 229–30
real-life considerations in, 243–58
relationships during, 249–52
support systems during, 226–28
technological aids for, 222–23
withdrawal symptoms during, 4–5
Rehabilitation, 79–80
Relapse
causes of, 231–32
chronic, 238
managing and recovering
from, 236–37
statistics on, 232
Relapse prevention
evaluating relationships for, 239–40
high-risk situations and, 237–39

managing and recovering
from slips, 236–37
preparing for, 231–35
self-esteem development for, 240–41
support systems for, 241–42
temptations and, 224–26, 234
trigger recognition and, 235–36
Relational addictions
chat room addiction, 159–60
cybersex, 157–59
danger of, 160
love addiction, 148–53
serial dating, 153–54
sex addiction, 154–57
talking to loved one about, 160–61
treatment for, 161–62
Relationships. *See also* Family
members/relationships
developing satisfying, 282–83
evaluating, 239–40
maintaining healthy, 251–52
Research, 29
Residential rehabilitation
programs, 80, 194, 195
Risk factors, 15–19
Ritalin, 73, 98
Role reversals, 267–70
R-rated movies, 41–42
Rush, Benjamin, 5, 27–28

Schools, 17–18
Secondhand smoke, 8, 88–89
Sedatives, 96
Selective serotonin reuptake
inhibitors (SSRIs), 126, 147, 173
Self-care, 275–78
Self-esteem, 17, 48, 150, 224, 240–41
Self-evaluation, 21–23
Self-help treatment options, 216
Self-pity, 242
Self-reflection, 274
Serial dating, 153–54
Serotonin, 50, 72, 73, 112–13,
137–38, 151–52
Serzone (nefazodone), 204
Sex addiction, 154–57
Sexual abuse, eating
disorders and, 110–11
Sexual paraphilias, 155–56
Shoplifting addiction, 131–33

Shopping/spending addiction, 123–26
Smoking. *See* Nicotine addiction
Smoking-cessation programs, 91–92
Snus, 83
Social costs, of gambling, 142–43
Social drinkers, 54–56
Social expectations, 43–44
Social learning, 33–34, 42, 45
Social pressure, x, 16–17, 111–12
Solitaire, 177
Spiritual direction, 278
Sponsors, 240
State-dependent learning, 60
State-sponsored gambling, 141–44
Steroids, 69
Stimulants, 68–69, 73, 74, 79, 96, 103–4
Substance abuse
vs. dependence, 1
overview of, 2–3
Substance addiction
categories of drugs for, 65–69
common substances of, 70–72
criminal element of, 75–76
overcoming, 78–79
rehab and recovery from, 79–80
signs and symptoms of, 74–75
talking to loved one about, 76–78
Substance dependence
vs. abuse, 1
overview of, 3–5
Sugar, 113
Suicide, 57
Support groups/systems, xi
for alcoholism, 28, 62–63, 216, 227
for food addiction, 119
for gambling addiction, 147
for nicotine addiction, 92
online, 222–23
for pornography addiction, 172
during recovery, 200, 226–28
for relapse prevention, 241–42
for relational addictions, 157, 162
for shoplifting addiction, 132
for substance addiction, 107
Synaptic gap, 6–7

Technological aids, for recovery, 222–23
Technological devices, 180–82
Technology addiction
anonymity and, 184–85

Technology addiction—*continued*
   cell phone addiction, 180–82
   dangers of, 175–76
   Internet addiction, 182–84
   overview of, 174–75
   talking to loved one about, 185–86
   treatment for, 186–87
   video game addiction, 177–80, 182
Teenagers. *See* Adolescents
Telemedicine, 224
Temptations, 43–44, 224–26, 234
Testosterone, 156
Therapeutic community (TC), 196
Therapy, 281
Thought distortions, 10–14, 219–20
Time management, 252–56
Tobacco products, 83, 89
Tolerance, 3–4, 5, 82
Topiramate (Topamax), 204
Tranquilizers, 96
Treatment, xi. *See also* Medications
   of alcoholism, 61–63, 203–05
   alternative, 209–16
   for behavioral addictions, 134–35
   budgeting for, 191–94
   choosing right, 194–97
   cognitive-behavioral therapy, 219–22
   costs of, 270–71
   denial as roadblock to, 188–91
   detoxification, 201–02
   faith-based, 216–17
   for food addiction, 118–19
   for gambling addiction, 146–47
   job consequences of, 198–99
   medications for, 203–9
   for nicotine addiction, 91–94
   for pornography addiction, 171–73
   for prescription drug addiction, 106–7
   professionals for, 197–98
   for relational addictions, 161–62
   risks of, 217
   seeking, 48
   for sex addiction, 157
   for shoplifting addiction, 132–33
   of substance addiction, 78–80
   talking to others about, 199–200
   for technology addiction, 186–87

Triggers, 47, 235–36
Trust, 271–72
Tryptophan, 50, 112–13, 114
Twelve-step programs, 62–63,
   80, 119, 147, 157, 172, 216

Ulcers, 52

Vaccines, addiction, 93, 205
Varenicline (Chantix), 206
Video game addiction, 42, 177–80, 182
Violence, video game, 180
Virtual reality, 184
Vitamin deficiencies, 53

Wernicke's encephalopathy, 53
Willpower, 27–28
Wine, 4
Withdrawal symptoms
   avoidance of, 4–5
   from depressants, 102
   detoxification and, 202
   from exercise addiction, 127
   from nicotine, 81–82, 86, 90
   from opiates, 101
   from stimulants, 104
   from substance addiction, 78–79
Women
   affect of alcohol on, 57–59
   prescription drug abuse among, 98
Woodward, Samuel, 28
Work addiction, 129–31

Yin/yang, 209
Yoga, 214
Youth. *See also* Children; Teenagers
   advertising aimed at, 40–41
   curiosity of, 41–43
   modeling behavior by, 45
   prescription drug abuse among, 98
Youth addiction, x, 16–18